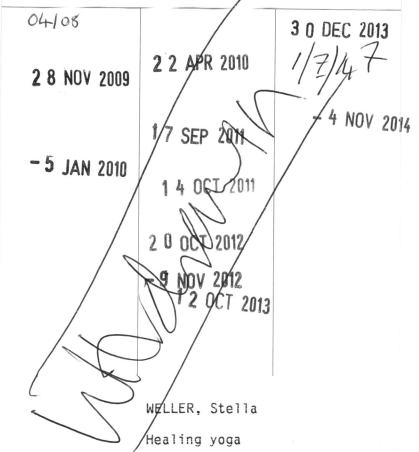

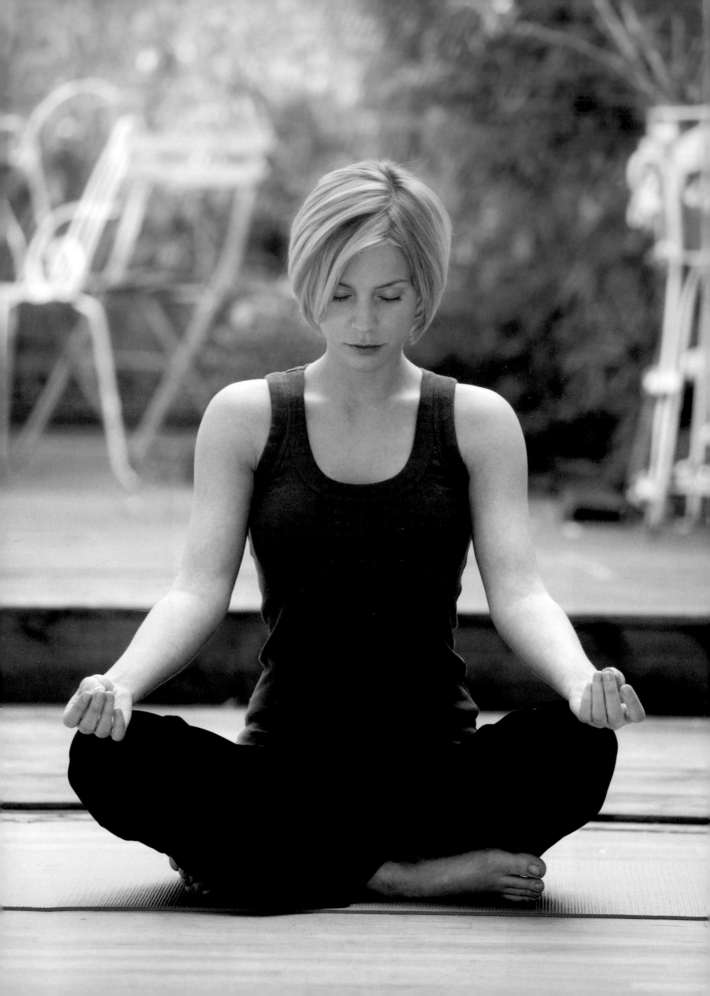

HEALING YOGA

Stella Weller

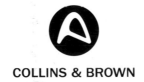

COLLINS & BROWN

CONTENTS

INTRODUCTION | 6

PART 1: GETTING STARTED | 12

PART 2: THE HEALING POWER OF YOGA | 28

Bones, muscles and joints | 30

Breathing and circulation | 50

Digestion and elimination | 66

Mental health | 78

Reproductive system | 94

Sleep and fatigue | 106

Metabolic disorders | 113

Immune system | 119

PART 3: WELLNESS ROUTINES | 124

INTRODUCTION

A doctor sets a broken bone or brings together the edges of a wound and secures them with sutures. Another doctor prescribes a medicine to halt the progression of a dreaded disease, but it is the body, not the doctor, that brings about the actual healing.

Regardless of the cause of damage, healing follows a predictable course that may be divided into four phases: vascular response, inflammation, proliferation and reconstruction. Within seconds of an injury, the body begins the first of these phases to control bleeding and limit the spread of infection. Blood vessels constrict, clotting begins and various protective and healing processes are set in motion. The other three phases follow the first in a beautifully synchronized fashion until the structure and function of the damaged tissues have been repaired and restored, and the equilibrium of the healing system has been re-established.

The healing system is composed of all the body's systems (such as the immune and nervous systems) and also of physiological components such as our mind and our breath. And when treatments work (such as those prescribed by a doctor), it is because they activate the healing mechanisms that are within us.

When we are injured or experience a breakdown in health, collaboration between us and our health-care provider (doctor or other qualified professional) usually offers the best chances of a satisfactory outcome. Therefore, let us not underestimate what we, as individuals, can do to contribute to this working relationship. For no matter where we are, we have within us (although often underutilized), natural resources that can promote health and healing: our body, our mind and our breath. These three components of the whole person have been part of the focus of the centuries-old discipline of yoga, and *Healing Yoga* will show you how to make them work for you – safely, efficiently and enjoyably.

More than 5000 years ago in India, a philosophy known as yoga came into being. The word "yoga" comes from Sanskrit and has various meanings, including "yoke" and "unity". It implies an integration of every aspect of the human being into a harmonious whole.

The principles of yoga were passed by word of mouth from master to student. About 3000 years later, an Indian sage named Patanjali finally recorded these teachings in a now-classical work called *Yoga Sutras*. This guidebook provided the framework for modern-day yoga practice.

The book has something to offer everyone, whatever their age or sex. Yoga can be very beneficial for pregnant women, but they should first seek permission from their doctor.

Health educators and fitness instructors will also find it a useful resource. And even if you are not recovering from an illness or injury, you can use the exercises and procedures to enhance your performance in sports, professional dancing and other activities, or to acquire stamina for increased productivity and fulfillment in any endeavour. Enjoy the exercises and savour their resulting health benefits.

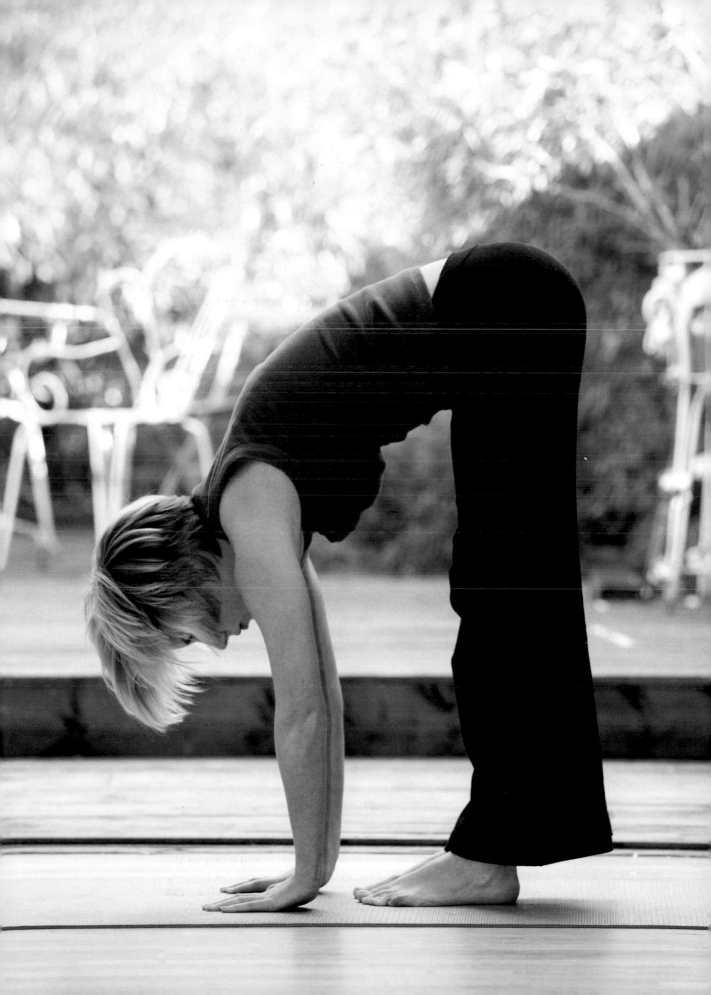

Tree of yoga

In ancient times, yoga was compared to a tree with six branches: bhakti, hatha, jñana, karma, raja and tantra. Each branch represented a particular approach to life. Most people in industrialized societies worldwide now practise hatha yoga. "Ha" means "sun" and "tha" means "moon".

Hatha yoga, then, may be considered a union of opposites to create balance. The system of hatha yoga (which will be referred to simply as yoga from now on) may be divided, for convenience, into five parts: asanas, pranayama, meditative practices, relaxation practices and cleansing practices.

1. Asanas

Generally regarded as physical exercises, yoga asanas are more accurately "poses comfortably held". They involve movements or series of movements by which muscle groups are put into action and energized. The manner in which this is done is economical: high levels of physical performance can be achieved with a minimal expenditure of energy.

Each asana involves the contraction of some muscle groups and the relaxation of their opposing muscles. Done slowly and with control, it heightens one's awareness of faulty postural habits and unnecessary muscle tensions.

Once the posture (exercise) has been completed, the practitioner is encouraged to visualize the beneficial effects, at first in the muscles and other structures on the outside of the body and then, in time, in the internal organs and tissues.

Each posture brings into action all the muscles and joints of a given part of the body. Consequently, muscles that tend to atrophy (waste away) through lack of regular exercise are now conditioned and receive an improved blood supply, while joints move freely as they lose their stiffness.

In many of the asanas, the vertebral column (spine) is subjected to gentle traction, thus releasing pressure on spinal discs and nerves. Increased spinal flexibility can lead to a reduction of pain and other discomforts, and posture is also improved.

The synchronized breathing required in the execution of all the exercises ensures good oxygen delivery to the working muscles. The full focusing of attention on the performance of the exercises has a tranquillizing effect on the nervous system, leading to a sense of calm and control.

These combined benefits, through regular practice over time, result in a strengthening of mind and body and a maintaining of wellness. Should health be disrupted, however, regular practice of the asanas will greatly contribute to reinforcing your healing system to help bring about recovery.

2. Pranayama

Exercises in voluntary breath control are collectively referred to as "pranayama". They take advantage of the fact that the respiratory (breathing) system is the only body system that is both involuntary and voluntary.

The primary function of the respiratory system is to provide oxygen for the body's metabolic needs and to remove carbon dioxide from the tissues. Respiration works very closely with circulation. It is through the circulation that tissues receive oxygen and nutrients, and the body is protected from agents of disease.

Because of the close collaboration between the respiratory and circulatory systems, techniques that train you to breathe efficiently will undoubtedly help you to function at your best when you are well. And when you are ill, they will maximize your chances of a satisfactory recovery by boosting your healing system.

The connection between breathing and feelings is undeniable. It is most noticeable when feelings are intense. In anger, for instance, breathing tends to be rapid and shallow, and in grief it may sound like a sob. In anxiety, particularly if it is marked, breathing can be so rapid as to border on hyperventilation (see page 50), with symptoms such as heart palpitations and feelings of lightheadedness.

During times of stress, or "fight or flight", breathing accelerates and the heart races in response to sympathetic nervous system activation. However, by wilfully slowing down your breathing you can help to elicit a parasympathetic nervous system response and a corresponding sense of calm.

Yoga trains you in acquiring and honing skills in voluntary attentive respiration, to help you to exert a measure of control over a function once thought to be involuntary only. This is highly empowering. It will equip you to cope with a wide variety of stressors, including pain and anxiety.

Yoga trains you to breathe efficiently, with minimum effort for maximum oxygen intake. And so when ill health occurs, this skill will enable you to maximize your healing potential.

3. Meditative practices

Meditation is a natural tool for relaxing your mind without dulling your awareness. Doctors refer to the meditative state as one of "restful alertness", which may seem to be a contradiction.

Simply put, when you are asleep, consciousness fades, oxygen consumption decreases and the heart rate becomes slower. When you are awake, by contrast, you are usually alert, oxygen consumption increases and your heart rate quickens. These opposite states are united during meditation, so that although you become deeply relaxed, you are nevertheless conscious and your mind is clear. A sense of peace ensues.

Meditative practices help to keep you in the present. States such as anxiety and depression, for example, represent concerns about and preoccupation with past and future events. Meditative practices help you to acquire a more reality-based perspective.

Meditation is also nature's tranquillizer. Unlike the chemical equivalents, it helps you to go deep within yourself to identify the source of disturbances and to bring them to the surface for more ready examination and resolution.

Most meditative practices make use of the breath as a focusing device (see the Humming Breath, page 48). Many of the exercises also employ visualization, or the ability to form mental pictures. This is done in a purposeful way, unlike daydreaming, which is usually unfocused and passive. Visualization can influence functions formerly believed to be outside the realm of voluntary control, such as heart rate, blood pressure and blood flow to various parts of the body. It can also help to speed up the healing of wounds, sore throat and a variety of other ailments.

Yoga meditative practices also utilize imagery, which includes the use of one or more of the senses such as touch, hearing and smell, in addition to visualization.

Imagery is sometimes used to prepare patients for certain medical procedures and to relieve pain and anxiety. For examples of the use of imagery, see the Pose of Tranquillity (page 62–63).

4. Relaxation practices

Relaxation is perhaps the most important prerequisite for healing any disorder. The muscles covering your body's bony framework (skeletal muscles) are rarely in a state of complete rest. They always retain a certain variable degree of tension. This is known as "basal tension" or "muscular tone".

Skeletal muscles, which are under voluntary control, have close links with internal structures by means of a nervous system network. Thus measures taken to reduce basal tension in the muscles can be effective in relaxing the internal organs. For example, a light massage of the abdomen can help to relieve pain or other discomfort in the stomach and intestines. This works by stimulating nerve endings at the body's surface and blocking the perception of pain. It also helps reduce muscle tension and spasm which intensify pain, and improve blood circulation and the elimination of waste products.

Another way of reducing basal tension in skeletal muscles is through gentle stretching exercises such as those of the yoga asanas. This works much like when a spring is stretched and then allowed to return to a resting state. Stretching muscles and briefly sustaining the stretch removes kinks and allows a free flow of blood for the delivery of oxygen and nutrients to the tissues. It also enhances lymph circulation to eliminate fatigue-producing substances. When the stretch is released, basal muscle tension is considerably reduced. Reducing basal tension in muscles conserves a great deal of otherwise wasted energy, thus combating fatigue and enhancing productivity.

Because muscular tension is influenced by psychological states, reducing it will have an impact on how you feel. For example, when you are anxious, muscles in various parts of your body, such as your face, jaw, neck, hands and lower back tighten unnecessarily. This increased muscle tension exerts pressure on underlying nerves and can generate pain and other discomforts. It also adds to the workload of the heart and lungs because breathing is inevitably affected.

One proven way of breaking this cycle of anxiety–tension–pain is through the use of your breath (see Pranayama, page 8–9).

Relaxation techniques

Local relaxation techniques target specific muscle groups in areas of the body where tension seems to gravitate and accumulate. Warm ups for the neck, shoulders, hands and ankles (see warm up exercises on pages 23–27) done periodically during the course of the day are very effective in decreasing basal muscle tension.

Systemic relaxation eliminates unnecessary tension from the whole body in a sequential and progressive manner. There is perhaps no better example of this type of relaxation than the time-honoured Pose of Tranquillity (Savasana), described in detail on pages 62–63.

5. Cleansing practices

Our body has the ability to eliminate various toxins through its excretory organs. These include: the urinary bladder and the kidneys, the colon, lungs and skin. The lachrymal (tear) ducts of the eyes also have excretory features, and when infected they can develop cysts and tumours.

Kriyas

Yoga traditionally included six purification practices, known as kriyas, to help the body get rid of accumulated poisons. They chiefly involved the respiratory system, the gastrointestinal system (stomach and intestines) and the eyes.

Because of their complexity, however, these hygiene practices have been modified for the convenience of today's practitioners. Apart from their usefulness in enhancing excretory functions, they help to strengthen tissues and prevent infection. They are useful complements to the other yoga techniques mentioned above.

For details of four of these procedures, please see Eye Splashing (page 122); Tongue Cleansing (page 122); Nasal Wash (pages 55 and 122); and Candle Concentration (page 65).

Yoga has become a highly respected and trusted discipline, not only by lay persons, but also, increasingly, by doctors and other health professionals. In fact, it forms the basis of many stress-reduction and health-promotion programmes. Physiotherapists and fitness instructors base many of their exercises on yoga, as do educators who prepare women for labour and childbirth.

Yoga Style

The yoga style that best typifies the practices presented in this book is "Viniyoga". Pioneered by the late T. Krishnamacharya and promoted by his son T.K.V. Desikachar, this style can most accurately be described as the art of personalized practice. Viniyoga is characterized by the adaptation of the exercises to suit the individual's needs and capabilities, rather than the individual conforming to the exercises. The asanas (postures) are done slowly and with awareness, and synchronized with regular breathing.

What yoga is not

There are still some uninformed individuals who equate yoga with religion. But although yoga developed alongside Hinduism and other religions, it has never been a religious practice. It is decidedly non-sectarian and is confidently practised by many people of various faiths. If you are still somewhat uncomfortable with the word, however, you may find it useful to think of yoga as a superb set of life skills to help you cope with stress, assist you in attaining optimal health and to help aid recovery if you have been ill.

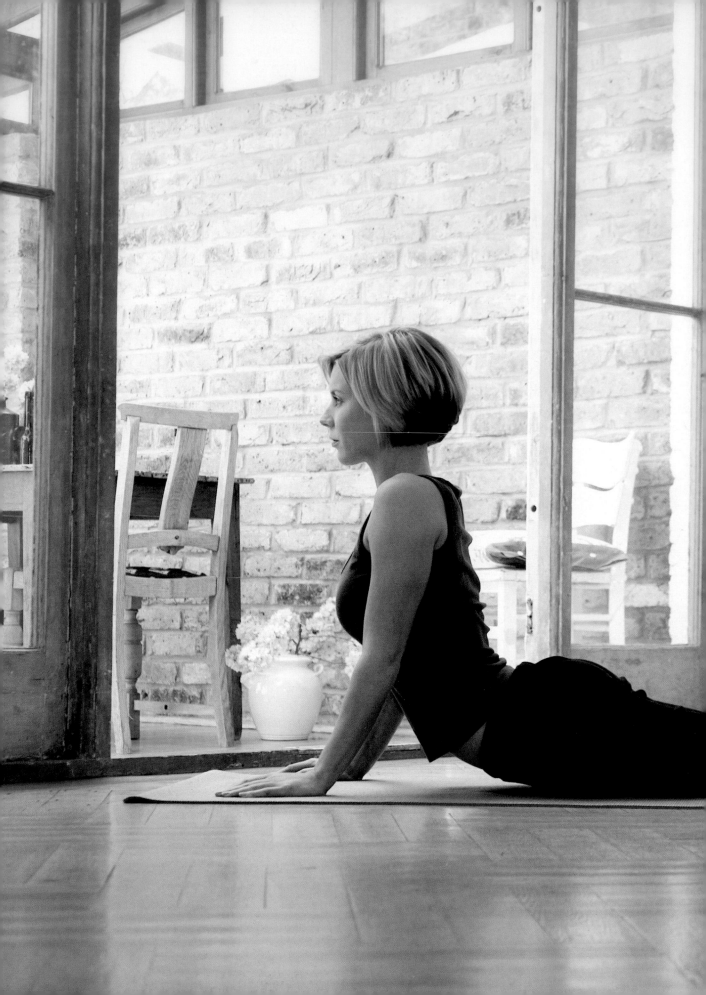

PART 1: GETTING STARTED

Equipped with an understanding of what yoga comprises and how to put its various disciplines into practice, you are now ready to embark on doing the exercises themselves. Set the scene by detaching yourself for a brief period of time from everyday concerns. Unite your physical resources with mental attributes such as your attentiveness and your ability to visualize, and with non-tangible components such as your breath and your belief in the infinite wisdom of the body's wonderful healing system.

Because you will probably be practising on your own, without supervision, the exercises and procedures in this book have been carefully selected with your safety in mind. Before attempting to do them, however, please check with your doctor or other professional health-care provider to be sure that the techniques are right for you to do.

How to use this book

The main part of the book is Part 2, The Healing Power of Yoga (pages 28–123), which is divided into sections that cover many common ailments and health problems. For each section, there are a number of recommended exercises to help bring relief and promote healing for those particular problems.

If you have a condition detailed in Part 2, please take a few moments to read about it, to help you to understand it or to refresh your memory. Then turn to the suggested exercises. With the permission of your doctor or other qualified health-care professional, try the regimen described, but by all means modify the exercises to suit your particular needs and level of functioning.

If you are in good health and wish to maintain it, please turn to Part 3 (page 124), which provides a number of routines, from five to 20 minutes duration, suitable for both men and women. Select one that you think will be compatible with your current schedule and other personal needs. Feel free to tailor your chosen routine according to your specific requirements. Whatever you decide to do, however, please plan to practise regularly: every day if you can, but at least every other day so as to obtain maximum benefit from your workout. Wherever possible, incorporate exercises into daily activities, at home or at the workplace. Some of the warm up exercises and some of the breathing exercises (such as the Anti-Anxiety Breath, page 60) are suitable for this purpose.

This section also has routines for women who are pregnant or have recently given birth. No matter what your state of health is, you will undoubtedly benefit from reading the background information in the Introduction (pages 6–11) and the rest of this chapter. It will enhance your appreciation of why yoga is so beneficial and how breathing, relaxation and cleansing practices work to promote your healing system.

Before attempting any of the exercises, it is vital that you read the Warming Up and Cooling Down routines (pages 22–27).

What to wear

To derive the greatest enjoyment from your yoga exercises, you need to feel comfortable. You must be able to move and breathe freely. Do not, however, wear garments that are so long and loose-fitting that they cause you to trip or in any way impede your movements. Long, loose hair may be a distraction. A ponytail that places pressure on your neck is best avoided.

Remove any items that may cause pressure, discomfort or injury, such as glasses, jewellery or a tight belt. When exercising during breaks at your workplace, loosen your clothing a little, to facilitate breathing and stretching. When relaxing after a workout, keep a light blanket, a sweater and pair of warm socks nearby in case you feel chilled.

Where to do it

One of yoga's attractions is that it can be practised in a variety of places, indoors or outdoors. Some techniques, such as breathing exercises (Pursed-Lip Breathing, page 54, for example) can even be done while travelling. Others can be practised where space is limited, such as the Infinity Neck Stretches (page 23), and yet others, such as the Pelvic Floor Exercise (page 77), can be done without those around you being aware of what you are doing.

Ideally, the place where you practise your exercises should be quiet and well ventilated. When performing at home, ask your family not to disturb you for the duration of your exercise session.

Practise on a level surface. If this is indoors, place a non-skid mat on a bare floor. This surface will be referred to as the "mat" in the exercise instructions.

When to do it

You can practise yoga at any time. You can integrate some of the exercises into your daily schedule, however busy, at home or at work. You can even practise some of the techniques when travelling or at the airport while waiting to board a flight.

You can do a few exercises on awakening in the morning to counteract stiffness of joints and to stimulate circulation. If you feel particularly stiff, taking a warm (not hot) shower or bath before practising your exercises may make it easier for you to stretch and bend. You can do a pre-sleep routine (see Sleep Disturbances, page 110) to promote refreshing slumber. For some people, practising before breakfast is the most convenient time. Others find that they need a glass of juice or a slice of toast to offset the low blood sugar level that exists after a night's sleep. In general, the best time to practise a session of yoga exercises is two to three hours after a meal, depending on its size and content. You may practise an hour after having a light snack.

If you have a specific yoga sequence you like, try to do it every day if possible. If this is not feasible, then certainly do it every other day so as not to lose the benefits gained from your previous practice session.

You may be more comfortable doing the exercises after emptying your bladder and perhaps your bowel, too. Some individuals also like to cleanse their tongue and nasal passages (pages 55 and 122) before doing a session of breathing exercises.

How to do it

A proper warm up before an exercise session is imperative to prevent strain and injury. Please see pages 22–27 for a selection of such exercises.

Precautions

As mentioned on page 14, if you are suffering from any medical condition or have health problems, please check with your doctor before attempting to do the exercises and procedures in this book.

You should not experience pain when doing an exercise. At the first hint of pain, stop. You may be doing the exercise incorrectly or it may not be an appropriate one for you to do at this time. In addition to the list below, please look out for other cautions and contraindications given in specific exercises.

• If you have had recent surgery, some of the exercises may not be suitable for you to do. Check with your doctor.

• When resuming exercise after a period of illness or inactivity, do so gradually. Consult your doctor or physiotherapist.

• If planning to do a vigorous workout just after waking up in the morning, make sure you warm up properly first. During sleep, spinal discs absorb extra fluid and so become more vulnerable than usual to compression and possible damage.

• If you are elderly or have been diagnosed with osteoporosis (pages 40–41), you may be prone to fractures if you fall. Be especially attentive and careful when doing balancing exercises, such as the Tree Posture (pages 42–43). Also, some forward-bending exercises like the Plough Posture (page 85) are contraindicated if you have osteoporosis, as they may result in compression fractures or other damage to spinal bones. Check with your doctor.

• If you have an ear or eye disorder, omit the practice of inverted postures, such as the Shoulderstand (page 84) and the Dog Stretch (page 58), which is also part of the Sun Salutation Series (pages 89–91). Also omit inverted postures if you have high blood pressure (page 61), a heart disorder or any condition that produces feelings of lightheadedness when you hang your head down.

• The inverted postures are also best omitted during your menstrual period.

• Avoid rapid abdominal breathing, as in the Dynamic Cleansing Breath (page 87) if you have a history of epilepsy, high blood pressure or heart disease.

• If you have a hernia, omit the Cobra (page 86), which is also part of the Sun Salutation Series (pages 89–91).

• If you have varicose veins or venous blood clots, avoid practising the Sun Salutation Series (pages 89–91); avoid staying in the Squatting Posture (page 45) and in seated folded-legs postures such as the Easy Pose (page 19) for any length of time.

Pregnancy

If you are pregnant, please check with your health-care provider (family doctor, obstetrician, midwife or physiotherapist) before attempting to practise any of the exercises in this book.

- Do not do the asanas during your first trimester (three months) if you have a history of miscarriage, actual or threatened. Do not do the Dynamic Cleansing Breath (page 87).

- Omit any exercise that feels awkward or uncomfortable.

- Omit exercises done in the prone position (lying on your abdomen), such as the Cobra (page 86).

- After the first trimester, avoid doing exercises that require you to lie flat on your back, such as the Bridge (page 38). This position can restrict the delivery of blood and oxygen to mother and foetus by placing pressure on the mother's vena cava (principal vein) and therefore draining the lower body.

The Asanas

Yoga asanas (postures, or physical exercises) are done slowly and attentively, in synchronization with regular breathing. Once a posture is completed, the position is held, for a varying period of time, according to the individual's comfort. The same slow, focused movement (or movements) is executed when coming out of the posture, again synchronized with regular breathing.

Staying focused while performing the asanas is emphasized. It ensures control of your position and movement at all times, and it helps to prevent injury.

Because of the awareness required when performing the asanas, they may be considered a sort of meditation in action. Meditative practices (pages 9–10) often incorporate breathing and imagery, as do the asanas. When you are in the holding phase of an exercise (indicated in the instructions as "hold"), do employ imagery with which you are comfortable. For example, when maintaining the Spinal Twist (pages 96–97), you may wish to visualize an increased blood flow to the kidney area, at the small of your back, bathing the adrenal glands and other nearby structures. You may also sense a comforting healing warmth in this part of the body.

Rest periods

A brief resting interval after each exercise is the usual practice. This period of relaxation is an important component of muscle activity. It helps to guard against stiffness and fatigue. A longer rest period, to cool down and recuperate, is generally taken at the end of an exercise session.

Counter postures

As a general rule, it is best to follow an exercise with a suitable counter posture. For example, after a backward-bending exercise such as the Camel (page 104), a forward-bending one such as the Pose of a Child (page 108) is a logical choice.

Breathing and meditation

The following points are worthy of note if you plan a session of breathing and meditation, separate from the asanas.

• Practise before, rather than directly after, a main meal. The process of digestion can interfere with concentration.

• Keep your body as relaxed as possible. Fidgeting detracts from the ability to stay focused. Make a quick top-to-toe check and consciously let go of unnecessary tension where you detect it.

• Unless otherwise instructed in a specific exercise, breathe in and out through your nose to warm, filter and moisturize the air on its way to the lungs. Keep your lips together but not compressed, and keep your jaw relaxed. Maintain a slow, even breathing rhythm, unless instructed differently. Do not hold your breath.

• You should sit still for several minutes to start with, and eventually up to 20 minutes. Here are three seated postures that will provide a comfortable seat and keep your spine properly aligned. They will also facilitate unrestricted breathing.

EASY POSE (SUKHASANA)

⊛ How to do it

1. Sit tall with your legs stretched out in front of you.
2. Fold one leg inwards and place the foot under the opposite thigh.
3. Fold the other leg and place the foot under the bent leg. Let the knees relax downwards naturally.
4. Rest your hands in your lap or on your thighs or knees. Relax your jaw and breathe regularly.

⊘ Notes

If at first you find it uncomfortable to sit as described above, try it sitting on a cushion.

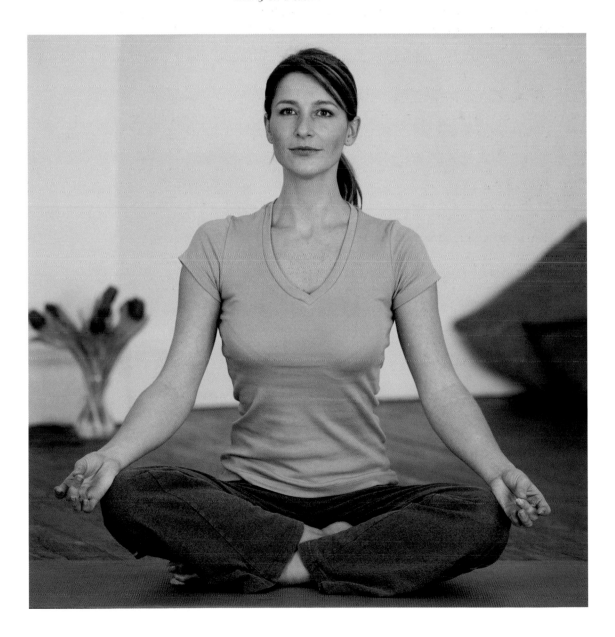

FIRM POSTURE (VAJRASANA)

⊛ How to do it

1. From a kneeling position with legs close together, lower your body to sit on your heels, Japanese style. Keep your trunk erect but not stiff, with the crown of your head uppermost.
2. Rest your hands on your thighs or knees. Relax your jaw and breathe regularly.

⊘ Notes

For greater comfort, you may insert a thin cushion or folded towel between your bottom and heels.

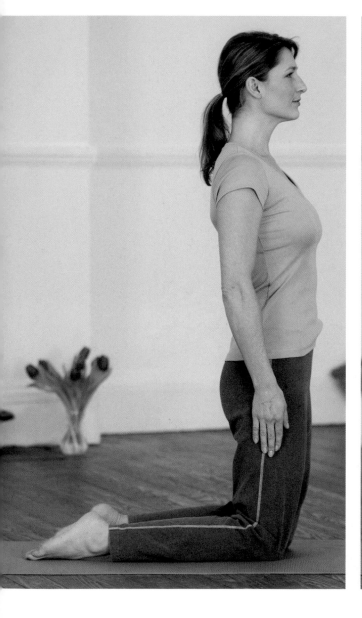
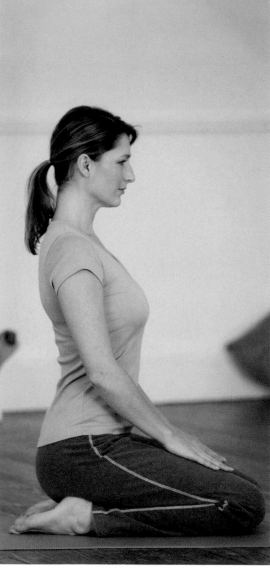

SITTING ON A CHAIR (MAITRIYASANA)

⊛ How to do it

1. Sit tall on a firm, straight-backed chair. Rest your feet flat on the floor.
2. Rest your hands on your thighs or knees. Relax your jaw and breathe regularly.

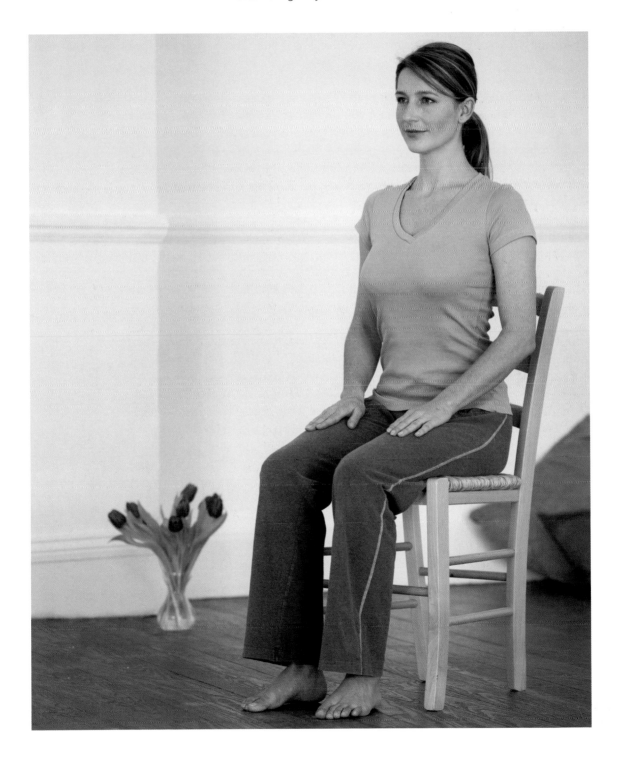

Warming up and cooling down

For the safe and effective practise of any exercise regimen, warming up before and cooling down after is imperative.

Warming up

Warm up exercises slightly increase body temperature, help to reduce stiffness and improve circulation. They are therefore useful in preventing the strain of muscles and joints once the main exercises are in progress. They are particularly important if you plan to do a vigorous workout early in the morning, shortly after a night's sleep. At this time, spinal discs are more vulnerable to compression and therefore to damage, since they will have absorbed extra fluid during the night. (As you move about during the day, the massaging action of the vertebrae reduces this fluid.)

Warm ups are also very important if you suffer from asthma. They help to avert the occurrence of bothersome symptoms that may arise during your workout.

Apart from the warm up exercises given on the following pages, you may also try the Sun Salutation Series (pages 89–91). Do them slowly and with awareness, and synchronized with regular breathing. Start with two sets and increase this number as you progress in your practice.

Cooling down

A cooling down period after your exercise session gives opportunity for static muscle stretching. This allows your cardiovascular system to return gradually to normal functioning. Problems such as feelings of dizziness and lightheadedness, which are symptoms of a sudden drop in blood pressure, may therefore be prevented.

Cooling down properly also enhances flexibility. In addition, it gives protection against drastic temperature changes in the lungs, which can constrict airways and induce asthma symptoms in susceptible individuals.

Many of the warm up exercises that follow may be done as cool down exercises, except the Rocking Horse (page 27). You may also wish to try the Sun Salutation Series (pages 89–91) for this purpose, but be sure to do them very slowly and attentively. Always maintain good posture when cooling down, to avoid incurring back strain. You may finish your exercise session, as many yoga students do, with the Pose of Tranquillity (page 62–63).

INFINITY NECK STRETCHES

⊕ What they do
▸ Keep the cervical (neck) part of the spine flexible and counteract stiffness.
▸ Contribute to a healthy spinal circulation.
▸ Prevent tension from building up in the neck.

⊛ How to do them
1. Sit tall in any comfortable position. Relax your shoulders, arms and hands. Close your eyes or keep them open. Relax your jaw and breathe regularly throughout the exercise.
2. Visualize the Infinity symbol (a figure-eight lying on its side). Trace its outline with your nose. Do this slowly and smoothly, five or more times. Pause briefly.
3. Repeat the exercise in the other direction five or more times. Rest.

⊘ Note
You may also do these stretches while standing.

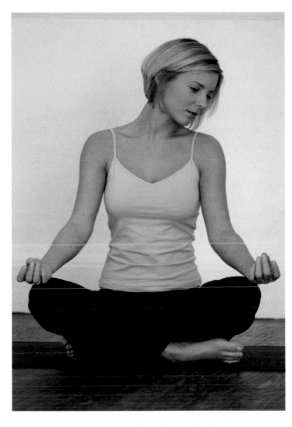

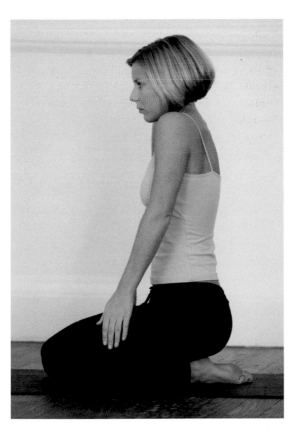

SHOULDER CIRCLES

⊕ What they do
▸ Enhance the effects of the Infinity Neck Stretches.
▸ Keep the shoulder joints freely moving and prevent stiffness.
▸ Improve circulation in the shoulders.
▸ Prevent a build up of tension in the shoulders.

⊛ How to do them
1. Sit or kneel in a comfortable position. Close your eyes or keep them open. Relax your jaw and breathe regularly throughout the exercise.
2. Draw imaginary circles with your shoulders in turn. Do so slowly and smoothly five or more times. Pause briefly.
3. Repeat the shoulder rotations five or more times in the opposite direction.

⊘ Note
You may also do this exercise while standing.

FIGURE-EIGHT WRIST ROTATIONS

⊕ **What they do**
▸ Keep hands, wrists and fingers supple.
▸ Improve circulation in these areas and strengthen them.
▸ Prevent tension from building up in the hands.

⊛ **How to do them**
1. Sit tall in any comfortable position. Close your eyes or keep them open. Relax your jaw and breathe regularly throughout the exercise.
2. Imagine a large figure-eight lying on its side in front of you. Trace its outline with open hands, slowly and smoothly, five or more times. Pause briefly.
3. Repeat the exercise in the opposite direction five or more times. Rest.

⊘ **Notes**
• *You may also do this exercise while standing or lying down.*
• *You may do it with one hand at a time.*

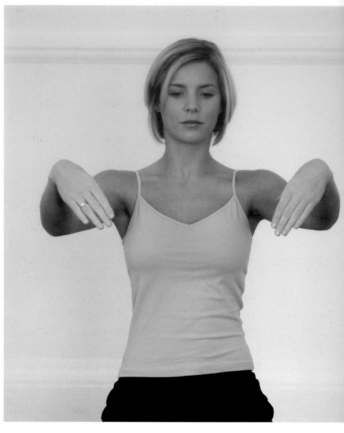

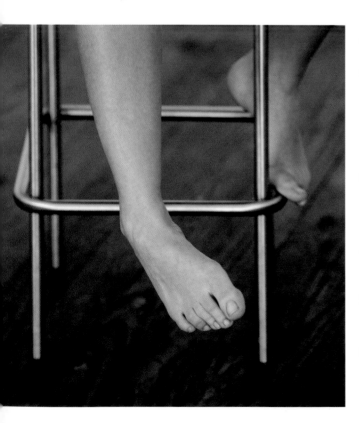

ANKLE CIRCLES

⊕ **What they do**
▸ Keep your ankle joints moving freely and prevent stiffness.
▸ Improve circulation in the feet.
▸ Help to strengthen the feet.

⊛ **How to do them**
1. Sit where you can move your feet freely. If sitting on the floor, lift and support one leg. Relax your jaw and breathe regularly throughout the exercise.
2. Draw imaginary circles with your foot or feet. Do this slowly and smoothly five or more times. Pause briefly.
3. Repeat the exercise in the other direction five or more times. Rest.

⊘ **Notes**
• *If rotating one ankle at a time, remember to do the same number of circles on each side.*
• *Can be done lying on your back, with one leg raised.*

BUTTERFLY

⊕ What it does

▶ Helps to keep the ankle, knee and hip joints moving freely and prevent stiffness.

▶ Stretches and tones the muscles of the inner thighs and groin.

▶ Improves circulation in the structures of the lower pelvis.

⊛ How to do it

1. Sit tall on your mat, with your legs stretched out in front. Relax your jaw and breathe regularly throughout the exercise.

2. Fold one leg inwards. Fold in the other leg and bring the soles of your feet together. Clasp your hands around the feet and bring them comfortably close to your body.

3. Rhythmically and at a moderate pace, alternately lower and raise your knees, like a butterfly flapping its wings. Do this from 10 to 20 times.

4. Carefully unfold your legs and stretch them out, one at a time. Rest.

ⓘ Caution

Omit this exercise if you have pain in you pubic area.

▽ Variation

1. Sit on your mat. Rest your palms on the mat beside your hips.

2. Fold your legs inwards, one at a time, and bring the soles of the feet together.

3. Alternately lower and raise your knees, from 10 to 20 times. in smooth succession.

4. Stretch out your legs and rest. Relax your arms and hands.

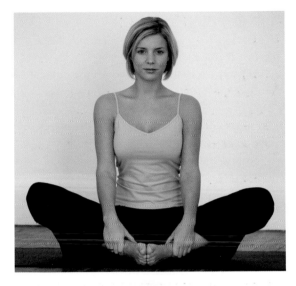

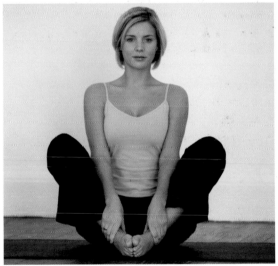

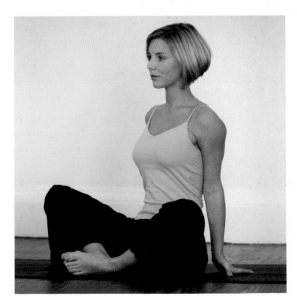

LYING PELVIC TWIST

⊕ What it does

▸ Stretches, strengthens and tones the oblique and transverse abdominal muscles and those of the lower back.
▸ Helps to keep the midriff trim.
▸ Facilitates mobility in the area of the diaphragm (between chest and abdomen).
▸ Promotes the health of pelvic structures.

⊛ How to do it

1. Lie on your back with your arms stretched sideways at shoulder level. Relax your jaw and breathe regularly.
2. Bend your legs, one at a time, and rest the soles of your feet on the mat. Bring your knees towards your chest.
3. Keeping your arms, upper body, and the small of your back in firm contact with the mat, exhale and tilt both bent knees together to one side.
4. Inhale and bring your knees, as a unit, back to the centre.
5. Exhale and tilt your knees to the other side.
6. Repeat the side-to-side tilting of your knees, from 10 to 20 times in smooth succession.
7. Resume your starting position. Rest.

▼ Variation

1. From a comfortable seated position, lean back on your elbows.
2. Bring your knees towards your chest.
3. Alternately tilt your knees, kept together, from left and right, synchronizing movement with breathing. Do this from 5 to 10 times in smooth succession.
4. Stretch your legs out and rest.

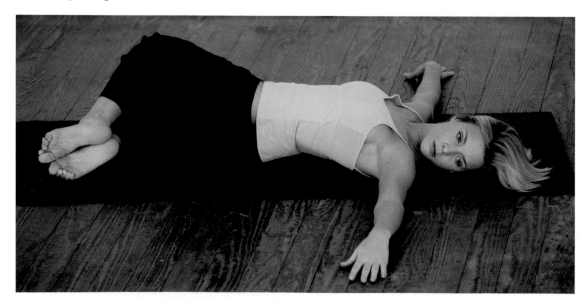

ROCKING HORSE

⊕ What it does

▸ Gently massages the back and helps to keep the spine flexible.

▸ Conditions the back and abdominal muscles.

▸ Loosens tight hamstring muscles (at the back of the legs). When these shorten, they affect the tilt of the pelvis and therefore posture.

⊛ How to do it

1. Sit on your mat with your legs out in front of you. Bend your legs and rest the soles of your feet flat on the mat, close to your bottom.

2. Pass your arms under your knees and hug your thighs. Make your back as rounded as you comfortably can. Relax your jaw and breathe regularly.

3. Inhale and kick backwards with both feet at once, to help you to roll onto your back.

4. Kick forwards on the exhalation following, to help you return to a sitting position. Avoid landing heavily on your feet so as not to jar your spine.

5. Repeat the back-and-forth rolling, five to eight times in smooth succession. Rest.

⚠ Caution

Omit this exercise if you are pregnant or have been diagnosed with osteoporosis. Check with your doctor.

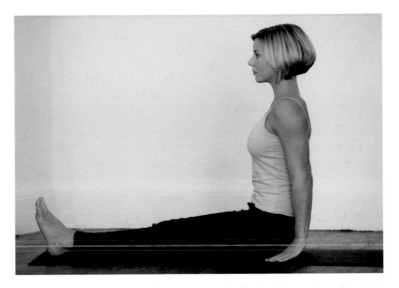

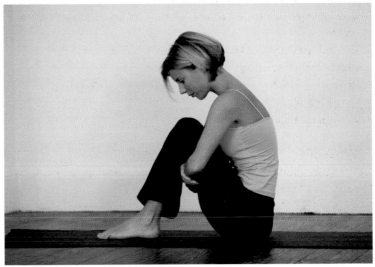

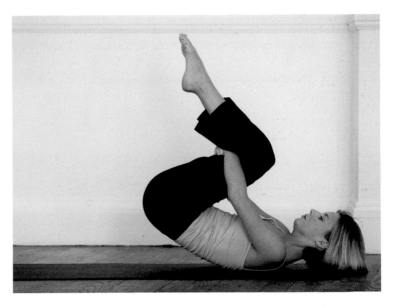

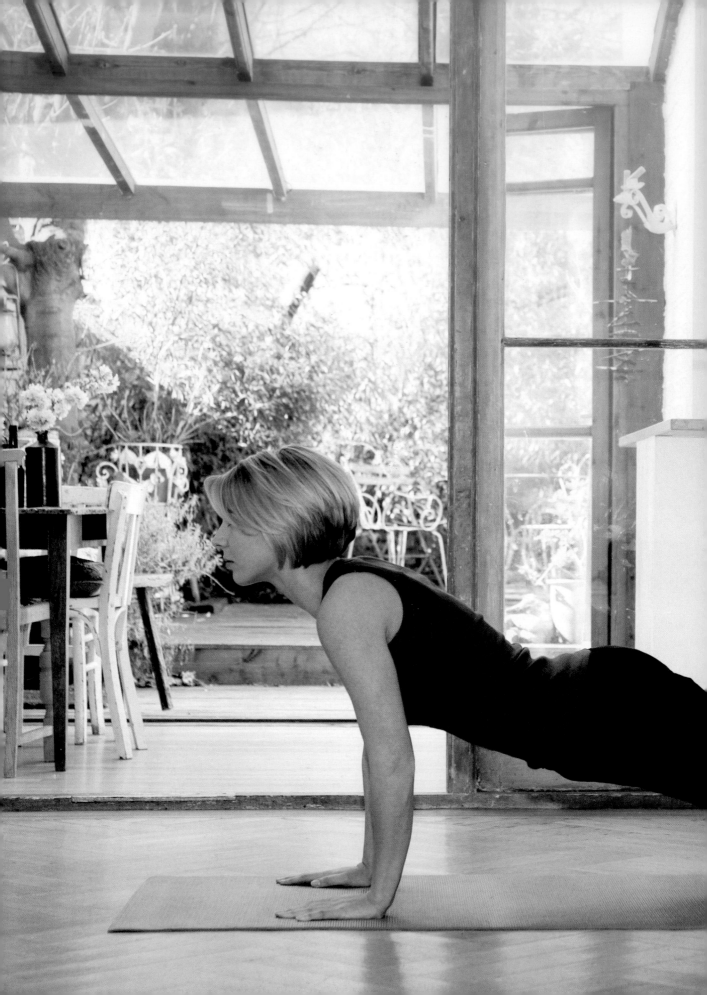

PART 2: THE HEALING POWER OF YOGA

The disorders presented in this section are among the most common and widespread. A brief overview of each is given, including its known or probable causes and its chief signs and symptoms.

Signs are manifestations of an illness. Symptoms are usually considered as changes in the body or its functions, which the person experiencing them perceives and may indicate disease or a phase of disease.

Along with background information on each disorder, selected exercises are given to help prevent it, to slow down its progression or to assist in its resolution and in the restoration of the body's normal functioning. The exercises will help to activate your own healing system. However, they are not to be regarded as a substitute for conventional medical care. It is imperative that you consult a qualified doctor or other health professional should you suffer any serious health problem.

You may find it useful, before attempting to do the exercises, to review Part 1 of the book to refresh your memory on the guidelines for safe practice, particularly the Precautions (pages 16–17).

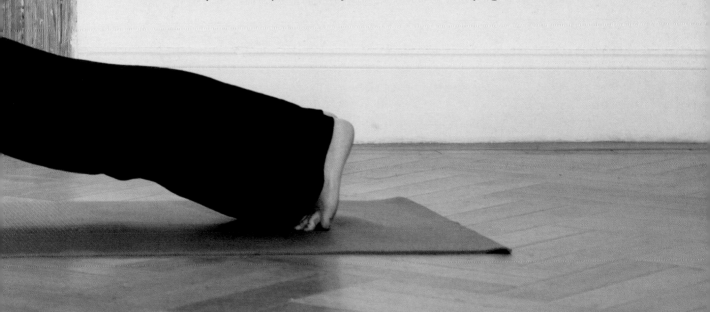

Arthritis

Arthritis literally means "joint inflammation". The word comes from the Greek "arthron", meaning joint, and "itis", meaning inflammation.

Arthritis describes an inflamed, stiff, swollen and sometimes painful joint, which is the consequence of a number of disease processes. The chief of these is inflammation.

There are more than 100 forms of arthritis. Some occur gradually as a result of normal wear and tear over time. Others appear suddenly and disappear just as suddenly. Yet others are progressive and become chronic.

Arthritis-like disorders can affect not only joints but also internal organs. Most of the causes underlying arthritis are unclear, but the following can contribute to its emergence: physical trauma such as a joint sprain; lack of physical activity; excessive body weight which places strain on joints; the ageing process; hormonal changes; genetic diseases that weaken cartilage (the protective and supportive tissue between bones and joints); immune system abnormalities; infectious agents such as viruses and bacteria; and emotional trauma.

Arthritis in its various forms may be associated with: cartilage breakdown as occurs in osteoarthritis (OA), rheumatoid arthritis (RA) and systemic lupus erythematosus (SLE); inflammation of the lining of joints (synovial membrane), muscles, blood vessels, tendons and ligaments; and loss of joint movement and decreased muscle strength.

Osteoarthritis (OA)

Also known as degenerative joint disease, OA is the most common form of arthritis. It affects women more than men. Related to the development of OA are obesity, excessive weight-bearing activities and high-impact sports, hormonal influences such as a decline in oestrogen production at menopause, and damage following fracture, surgery or infection. OA chiefly affects the larger weight-bearing joints, such as the hips and knees.

Rheumatoid Arthritis (RA)

RA is the most common type of inflammatory arthritis. Women tend to develop RA in their thirties and forties, and men in their fifties and sixties. There appears to be a genetic predisposition to RA, and hormonal fluctuations also seem to play a part. For example, symptoms tend to abate during the last trimester (three months) of pregnancy but to flare up following childbirth.

RA can appear because the normal functioning of the immune system has been disturbed. The concept of RA as an autoimmune disease, in which the body literally turns against itself, is currently in question.

In RA, the joints mostly affected are those of the fingers, hands and wrists initially, and later the larger joints such as the knees and hips.

Ankylosing spondylitis

This term comes from the Greek words "ankylos", meaning crooked, and "spondylos", meaning vertebra. Ankylosing spondylitis is a condition in which not only spinal joints are inflamed, but also tendons and ligaments where they attach to spinal bones. This form of arthritis usually occurs in men before the age of 40. As it progresses, it can result in a forward flexion of the spine, commonly referred to as a "poker" or "bamboo" spine. Although there is a strong hereditary component, the exact cause of the disorder is unknown.

In addition to involving the spine, ankylosing spondylitis can affect the hips, shoulders, neck, ribs and jaw. It can also affect the joints where ribs meet vertebrae and so make breathing difficult.

The most prominent feature of this disorder is lower back pain that persists for at least three months, and which improves with exercise but not with rest. Other manifestations are decreased mobility of the lumbar spine, reduced chest expansion, and inflammation of the sacroiliac (sacrum and pelvis) joints.

Systemic lupus erythematosus (SLE)

SLE is an inflammatory condition that affects numerous parts of the body. Generally, however, there is no damage to bone or cartilage. It mostly occurs in women of reproductive age, first appearing between 15 and 25 years.

The specific causes of SLE, although not fully known, appear to be a combination of genetic and environmental factors. SLE is often considered an autoimmune disorder, in which the body attacks rather than defends itself. Adverse reactions to some drugs may also produce lupus-like symptoms.

Signs and symptoms of SLE, which can be numerous, include a skin rash ("butterfly rash") over the nose and cheeks, weakness and fatigue, weight loss, sensitivity to light and hair loss.

FIGURE-EIGHT WRIST ROTATIONS

⊕ What they do
▸ Keep hands, wrists and fingers supple.
▸ Improve circulation in these areas and strengthen them.
▸ Prevent tension from building up in the hands.

⊛ How to do them
1. Sit tall in any comfortable position. Close your eyes or keep them open. Relax your jaw and breathe regularly throughout the exercise.
2. Imagine a large figure-eight lying on its side in front of you. Trace its outline with open hands, slowly and smoothly, 5 or more times. Pause briefly.
3. Repeat the exercise in the opposite direction five or more times. Rest.

⊘ Notes
• *You may also do this exercise while standing or lying down.*
• *You may do it with one hand at a time.*

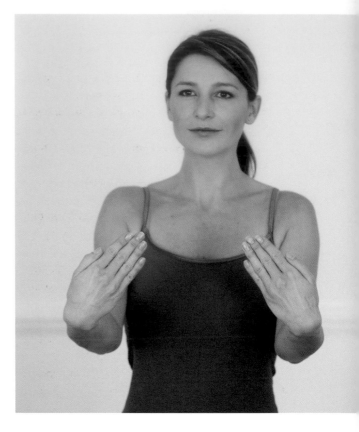

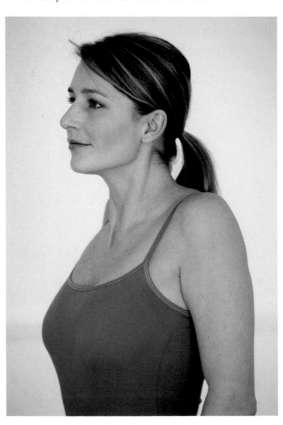

SHOULDER CIRCLES

⊕ What they do
▸ **Enhance the effects of the Infinity Neck Stretches.**
▸ **Keep the shoulder joints freely moving and prevent stiffness.**
▸ **Improve circulation in the shoulders.**
▸ **Prevent a build up of tension in the shoulders.**

⊛ How to do them
1. Sit tall in any comfortable position. Close your eyes or keep them open. Relax your jaw and breathe regularly throughout the exercise.
2. Draw imaginary circles with your shoulders. Do so slowly and smoothly five or more times. Pause briefly.
3. Repeat the shoulder rotations 5 or more times in the opposite direction.

⊘ Note
You may also do the Shoulder Circles while standing.

BUTTERFLY

⊕ What it does

▸ Helps to keep the ankle, knee and hip joints moving freely and prevents stiffness.

▸ Stretches and tones the muscles of the inner thighs and groin.

▸ Improves circulation in the structures of the lower pelvis.

⊛ How to do it

1. Sit tall on your mat, with your legs stretched out in front. Relax your jaw and breathe regularly throughout the exercise.

2. Fold one leg inwards. Fold in the other leg and bring the soles of your feet together. Clasp your hands around the feet and bring them comfortably close to your body.

3. Rhythmically and at a moderate pace, alternately lower and raise your knees, like a butterfly flapping its wings. Do this from 10 to 20 times.

4. Carefully unfold your legs and stretch them out, one at a time. Rest.

① Caution

Omit this exercise if you have pain in your pubic area.

▽ Variation

1. Sit on your mat. Rest your palms on the mat beside your hips.

2. Fold your legs inwards, one at a time, and bring the soles of the feet together.

3. Alternately lower and raise your knees, from 10 to 20 times, in smooth succession.

4. Stretch out your legs and rest. Relax your arms and hands.

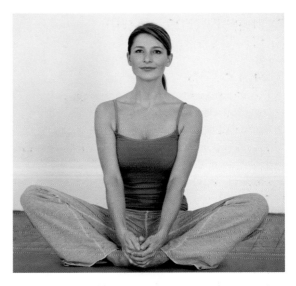

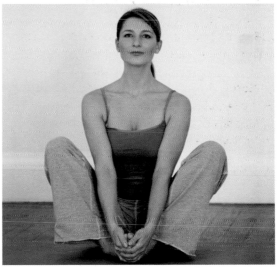

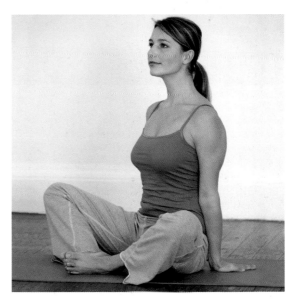

COW HEAD POSTURE (GOMUKHASANA)

⊕ **What it does**
▸ Helps to keep the arm and shoulder joints moving freely and prevent stiffness.
▸ Facilitates deep breathing.
▸ Counteracts the possible ill effects of too much forward bending.
▸ Encourages good posture.

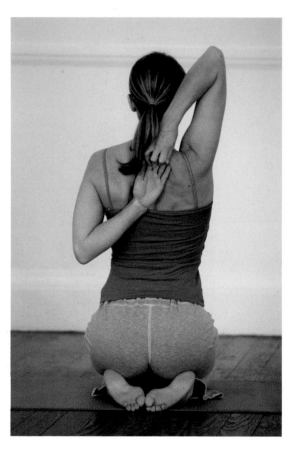 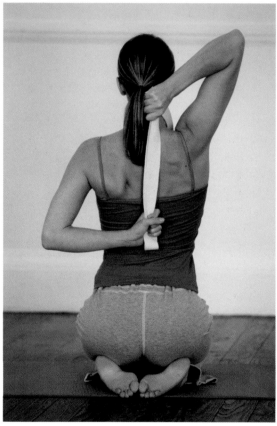

⊛ **How to do it**
1. Stand or sit in any comfortable position. Relax your jaw and breathe regularly.
2. Reach over your right shoulder with your right hand. Keep your arm near your ear and point your elbow upwards.
3. With your left hand, reach behind you from below and interlock your fingers with those of your right hand. Maintain good posture.
4. Hold this posture for five to 10 seconds and keep breathing regularly.

5. Relax your arms.
6. Repeat the exercise with the arm positions reversed.
7. Shrug your shoulders a few times. Rest.

⊘ **Notes**
If you are not able to interlock your fingers, use a scarf, belt or other prop. Toss one end over your shoulder, grasp the other end from below and gently pull the two hands apart.

EAGLE POSTURE (GARUDASANA)

⊕ What it does
▸ Provides gentle exercise for all the joints of your arms and legs, to keep them moving freely and to prevent stiffness.
▸ Helps to improve concentration, nerve-muscle coordination and alertness.

⊛ How to do it
1. Stand tall, with your arms at your sides. Relax your jaw and breathe regularly throughout the exercise.
2. Shift your weight onto your left foot. Carefully lift your right foot and cross your right leg over your left; hook the toes around the lower left leg, if you can, without exerting unnecessary pressure. Keep your body as erect as possible.
3. Bend your arms and place one within the other in front of you. Rotate your wrists until your palms are together.
4. Hold the posture for as long as you comfortably can while breathing regularly.
5. Carefully resume your starting position. Rest briefly.
6. Repeat the exercise, reversing the position of the arms and legs.

⊘ Notes
• *To help you to stay steady, focus your attention on your own regular breathing or fix your gaze on a still object in front of you, such as a door handle.*
• *When first trying this posture, stand near a post or wall and use it to help you maintain your balance.*

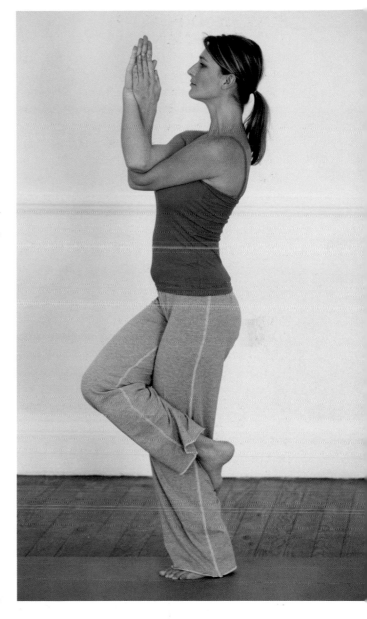

DIVIDED BREATH

⊕ What it does
▸ **Relaxes tense chest muscles and facilitates deep breathing.**
▸ **Allays anxiety and promotes calm.**

⊛ How to do it
1. Sit tall in any comfortable position. Relax your jaw. Relax your hands and any other obviously tense body parts.
2. Take two, three or more short, inward breaths, as if breaking up an inhalation into equal parts.
3. Exhale slowly and steadily through your nose, or through pursed lips as if cooling a hot drink.
4. Repeat steps 2 and 3: divided inhalation followed by steady exhalation through nose or mouth, until you feel your chest relaxing and you can then take one comfortable deep inward breath.
5. Resume regular breathing.

Back problems

About 80 percent of us will, at some time in our lives, experience back pain or a back-related problem.

The spine provides a support for the head and trunk, and also serves as a point of attachment for the ribs, pelvis and back muscles. Although it is strong and flexible it is nevertheless vulnerable to and affected by a myriad of disorders. Common conditions include disc problems, notably a herniated ("slipped") disc; various forms of arthritis, such as osteoarthritis (page 30) and ankylosing spondylitis (page 31); numerous injuries such as fractures; osteoporosis (page 40); scoliosis (lateral curvature of the spine); tumours in any part of the body, such as the uterus and prostate gland; infection, and even the effects of hormonal changes, such as those occurring in pregnancy.

Spinal health can also be influenced by factors such as weight gain or loss, stress, inactivity and poor postural habits.

Preventive measures

We can, however, do a great deal more than we may have previously believed to prevent certain back problems from arising. Important preventive measures include habitually practising correct body mechanics, that is, being careful about the way in which we use our body and its various parts in everyday activities. Performing stretching and strengthening exercises every day can also help to alleviate the pain of back problems. Being too busy should not deter you from doing so because you can inconspicuously integrate a number of such exercises into your daily schedule at home or in your workplace.

Even when back pain or any other back-related problem strikes, experts agree that we can do more as individuals to bring relief and help to restore function than any other single measure, surgical or non-surgical, can achieve.

CURL UP (YOGA SIT UP)

⊕ What it does

▶ Strengthens the rectus abdominus muscles (which run up and down the front of the abdomen), and so provides reinforcement for the muscles supporting the spine and pelvis. (Weak abdominal muscles are a common cause of backache.)

▶ Keeps the spine flexible.

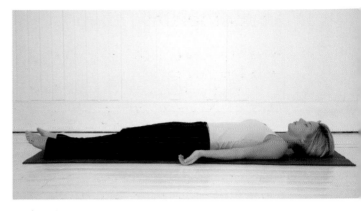

⊛ How to do it

1. Lie on your back with your legs stretched out in front and slightly separated. Relax your jaw and breathe regularly.

2. Bend your knees and slide your feet towards you until the soles are flat on the mat. Maintain this distance between feet and body. Rest your palms on the tops of your thighs.

3. Exhale and carefully raise your head. Fix your gaze on your hands as you slide them towards your knees. Stop when you feel the maximum tolerable tension in your abdomen.

4. Hold the posture for as long as you comfortably can while breathing regularly.

5. Slowly and smoothly curl yourself back onto your mat as you inhale.

6. Relax your arms and hands at your sides. Stretch out your legs and rest while breathing regularly.

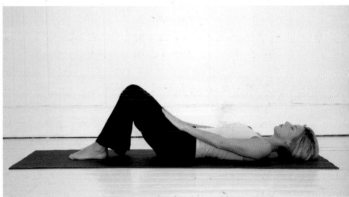

▽ Variation

1. Follow steps 1 and 2 from above.

2. As you exhale, slowly and carefully lift your head and then curl your body forwards. Stretch your arms and reach towards the outside of your left knee.

3. Hold the posture for as long as you comfortably can while breathing regularly.

4. Inhale and curl yourself back onto the mat. Stretch your legs out. Relax your arms at your sides. Rest briefly while breathing regularly.

5. Repeat steps 2 to 4, this time reaching for the outside of your right knee.

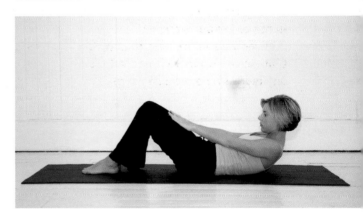

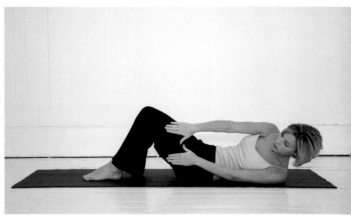

BRIDGE (SETU BANDHA)

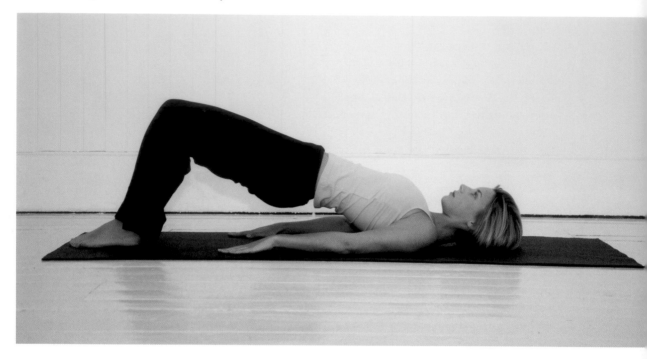

⊕ What it does
▸ Tones the muscles at the front and back of the body.
▸ Helps to keep the spine flexible.

⊛ How to do it
1. Lie on your back with your legs stretched out in front and your arms beside you. Relax your jaw and breathe regularly.
2. Bend your legs and rest the soles of your feet flat on the mat, a comfortable distance from your bottom. Turn your palms down.
3. Inhale and slowly and smoothly raise your back from the mat, first lifting your hips, followed by your lower and finally your upper back. Avoid arching your spine.
4. When you have reached your comfortable limit, hold the posture for as long as you can, with ease. Keep breathing regularly.
5. To come out of the posture, lower your back in a smooth and connected manner, starting with your upper back. Visualize lowering one vertebra at a time.
6. Stretch out, as in your starting position, and rest.

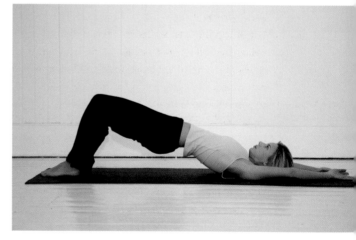

▼ Variation
1. For a more intense stretch, follow the instructions for the basic Bridge, above. Then stretch your arms overhead.
2. Hold the posture for as long as you comfortably can while breathing regularly.
3. To come out of the posture, bring your arms back to the sides of your body, then slowly lower your torso starting with your upper back, then lower back and hips. Stretch out your legs and rest.

KNEE HUG (VATAYANASANA)

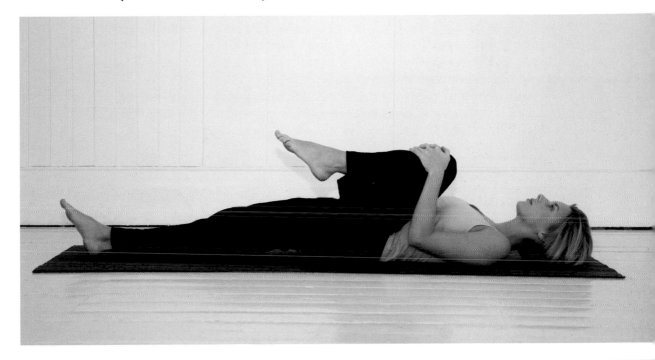

⊕ What it does
▸ Tones the back and abdominal muscles.
▸ Relaxes the back and relieves minor backaches.
▸ Helps to expel gas from the stomach and
  intestines.

⊛ How to do it
1. Lie on your back with your legs stretched out in
   front and arms at your sides. Relax your jaw and
   breathe regularly.
2. On an exhalation, bend one leg and bring the
   knee towards your chest. Hold it in place with
   your hands.
3. Maintain the posture for as long as you
   comfortably can while breathing regularly.
4. Return to the starting position.
5. Repeat the exercise with the other leg. Rest.

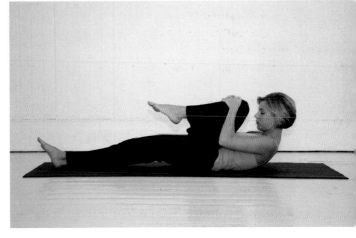

▼ Variation
1. Follow the instructions for the basic Knee
   Hug, above.
2. Very carefully lift your head and bring your
   forehead towards the bent knee.
3. Hold the posture for as long as you comfortably
   can while breathing regularly.
4. Return to the starting position.
5. Repeat the exercise with the other leg.

Osteoporosis

The word "osteoporosis" means "porous bones". It describes a disease process that weakens bones and makes them brittle and prone to fracture. In some cases, bones that were once dense and strong could be so affected that even normal stresses such as bending over or twisting the torso could result in injury.

The most serious loss of bone occurs in the spine and femur (thigh bone). The spinal bones (vertebrae) may become compressed by the weight of the body itself once weakened by osteoporosis. Compression fractures can actually reduce one's height by several centimetres.

Osteoporosis affects mainly postmenopausal women and, to a lesser extent, sedentary men. The foundation for the disorder is frequently laid in early adulthood. When young women, in particular, limit their food intake to control their weight, they often fail to get an adequate supply of calcium and vitamin D, so crucial in the teens and early twenties. It is at this age that eating disorders tend to occur.

Clinical manifestations of osteoporosis include shortened stature; difficulty in bending over; marked kyphosis ("dowager's hump"); impaired breathing (due to spinal and ribcage deformities); back pain; oral and dental problems, due to bone loss in the jaw bone.

Once osteoporosis occurs, treatment tends to be less than satisfactory. Therefore the key to successfully dealing with this disorder is to identify those individuals who are at early risk and take effective measures to prevent it.

Osteoporosis risk – non-modifible factors:

- **Age**
  Women past menopause and both women and men of advanced age are most at risk. When women enter menopause, the production of the hormones oestrogen and progesterone declines. These hormones stimulate the formation of new bone.

- **Heredity**
  Heredity influences bone mass. A family history of osteoporotic fracture is therefore useful in assessing a person's risk of developing the disorder.

- **Reproductive factors**
  Low bone mass is often associated with women who have had few pregnancies and irregular menstrual periods.

- **Race**
  Women of Hispanic descent, Caucasian women of very fair complexion and Asian women have a greater risk of developing osteoporosis.

- **Body build**
  Thin, small-boned individuals who also have low body weight are more susceptible to osteoporosis than those who are more sturdily built.

Modifiable risk factors:

- **Habits**
  Such as smoking cigarettes, drinking alcohol in excess, malnutrition, lack
  of regular exercise and the use or misuse of certain medicines are among the
  changeable risk factors.

- **Smoking**
  Experts believe that tobacco is toxic to bone and that it may also contribute to
  decreased oestrogen levels.

- **Alcohol**
  Drinking alcohol in excess can be directly or indirectly toxic to bone. Heavy
  drinkers, in fact, tend to receive most of their calories from alcohol rather
  than from a nutritious diet.

- **Diet**
  A diet that is deficient in protein, calcium and vitamin D, and too high in
  phosphorus, is not conducive to bone health.

- **Exercise**
  Exercise subjects bones to a certain amount of stress, and bones respond by
  strengthening themselves. Exercise also improves muscle strength and tone,
  both of which are necessary for healthy bones.

- **Medications**
  Prolonged use of some medicines may adversely affect the integrity of bone. They
  include: antacids containing aluminum, which accelerate the excretion
  of calcium; diuretics ("water pills"), some of which promote calcium loss; some
  laxatives, particularly mineral oil, which depletes stores of vitamins A, D, E and K;
  steroids, often used to treat inflammatory diseases such as arthritis, as they may
  inhibit bone formation and, over time, decrease muscle mass (the pull of muscles
  is important for bone mass and strength), and also lower oestrogen and
  testosterone levels and inhibit calcium absorption.

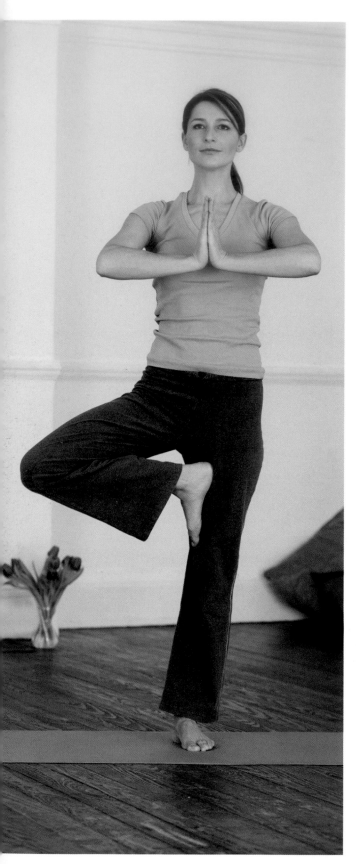

TREE POSTURE (VRIKSHASANA)

⊕ What it does
▶ Strengthens the leg muscles.
▶ Improves nerve–muscle coordination.
▶ Improves balance, alertness and concentration.

⊛ How to do it
1. Stand tall with your arms at your sides. Relax your jaw and breathe slowly and smoothly throughout the exercise.
2. Carefully shift your weight onto your left foot. Bend your right leg and use your hands to help you place the sole of the foot against the inner left thigh, as high up as is comfortable.
3. Bend your arms and put your palms together in front of your chest, in "prayer" or "namaste" position (see page 89).
4. Hold the posture as long as you can while breathing regularly.
5. Relax your right leg and resume your starting position, using your hands to help if necessary. Rest briefly.
6. Repeat the exercise standing on the right foot. Rest.

⊘ Notes
- *When first trying to do the Tree Posture, you may stand near a post or wall. Hold on to it to steady youself, if necessary.*
- *To help you maintain balance, rivet your attention on your own regular breathing, or fix your gaze on a still object in front of you, such as a picture on a wall or a door handle.*

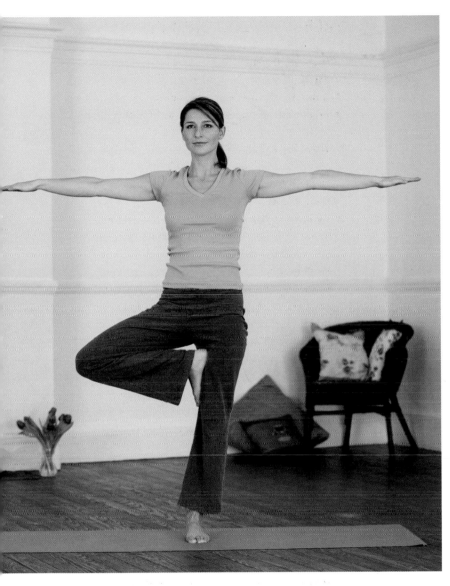

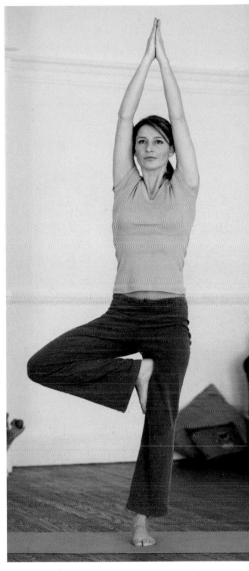

⬤ Variations

Try varying the position of the arms. Stretch them straight overhead and bring your palms together if you can, somewhat like a coniferous tree. Or stretch your arms sideways, like the branches of a spreading chestnut tree.

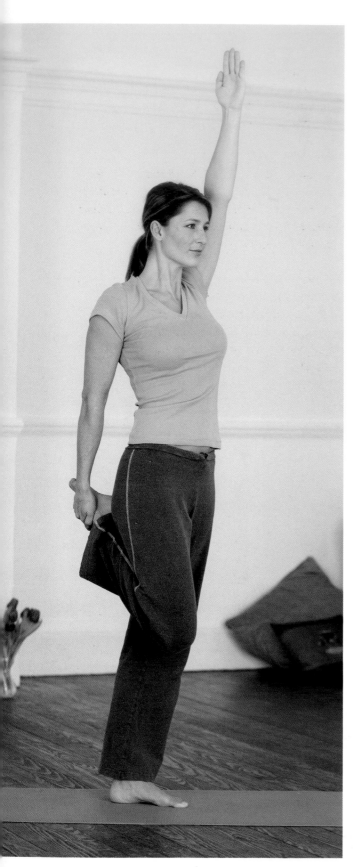

BALANCE POSTURE (QUADRICEPS STRETCH)

⊕ What it does

▸ Strengthens the legs.

▸ Conditions the powerful quadriceps muscles of the thighs.

▸ Improves balance, nerve–muscle coordination, concentration and alertness.

⊛ How to do it

1. Stand tall with your arms at your sides. Relax your jaw and breathe regularly throughout the exercise.
2. Carefully shift your weight onto your left foot. Bend your right leg backwards, and with your right hand bring the foot as close to your bottom as you comfortably can. Raise your left arm straight up above your head.
3. Hold the posture as long as you can while breathing regularly.
4. Relax your arms and leg and resume your starting position. Rest briefly.
5. Repeat the exercise standing on your right foot. Rest.

⊘ Notes

• *When first trying to do this exercise, you may stand near a wall or post. Hold on to it to steady yourself, if necessary.*

• *To help you maintain balance, rivet your attention on your own regular breathing, or fix your gaze on a picture on a wall or on a door handle, or some other still object infront of you.*

SQUATTING POSTURE

⊕ What it does
- Relieves pressure on spinal discs through gentle traction of the spine.
- Improves spinal flexibility.
- Tones back, abdominal and pelvic floor muscles.
- Strengthens ankle, knee and hip joints and keeps them moving freely; prevents stiffness.
- Useful in counteracting constipation.

⊛ How to do It
1. Stand with your feet comfortably apart and arms at your sides. Relax your jaw and breathe regularly throughout the exercise.
2. Slowly lower your body as if to sit on your heels. Keep your feet flat.
3. When you have reached your comfortable limit, hold the posture for as long as you can, but keep breathing regularly. Arrange your arms and hands for maximum comfort.
4. Slowly come out of the posture to resume your starting position. Rest.

▽ Variation
Instead of holding the posture, alternate between squatting and standing up, several times in smooth succession.

⊘ Note
Integrate squatting into daily activities. Squat to dust the lower parts of furniture or to tidy the contents of a bottom drawer. Squat to retrieve an object dropped on the floor, rather than bend over to do so. Squat to pull up weeds in your garden.

⊙ Caution
This posture, in its static version, is not recommended if you have varicose veins or venous blood clots. You may, however, alternate between going into the posture and standing up again. But first check with your doctor.

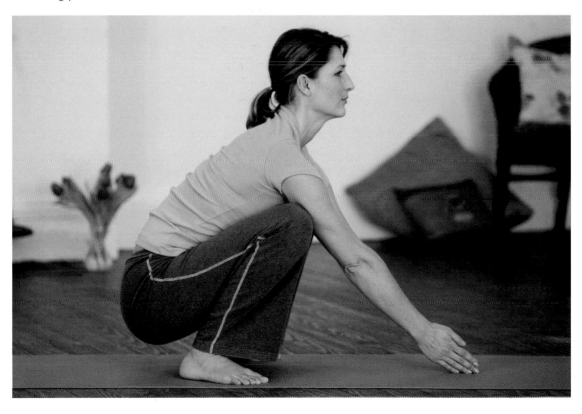

Repetitive Strain Injury (RSI)

Repetitive Strain Injury (RSI) refers to a group of disorders that predominantly affect the neck, shoulders, arms, elbows, wrists, hands and fingers. As the name suggests, it is usually brought on or worsened by repetitive activity over a long period of time. It is also known as: Repetitive Stress Injury, Cumulative Trauma Disorder, and Occupational Overuse Syndrome. It is a common problem in our high-tech world. RSI affects a number of body tissues, in particular the ligaments, muscles, nerves, tendons and synovial tendon sheaths.

Researchers have identified a number of factors which they believe contribute to the development of RSI. These include: repetitive activity, fatigue, pace of work, vibration, awkward static postures, unrelieved long-term activity, equipment design, high-pressure working environment, lack of regular exercise, poor nutrition, smoking and being overweight.

Medical conditions that make you more vulnerable to RSI include diabetes and arthritis (page 30).

Carpal Tunnel Syndrome (CTS)

One example of RSI is the well-known Carpal Tunnel Syndrome (CTS). This is a disorder of the wrist and hand. It is induced by compression on the median nerve, which supplies the palm and the thumb side of the hand.

Symptoms of CTS

Weakness of the hand and loss of power in the grip, so that there is a tendency to drop objects; burning, tingling or aching that sometimes radiates to the forearm and shoulder; muscle wasting due to not using the affected parts because of pain, and which consequently affects thumb and finger dexterity. The pain may be so intense that it may interfere with sleep.

Preventing RSI

Prevention is undoubtedly the best approach to dealing with what has become a widespread problem. Try to create a comfortable work environment designed to fit your individual needs and be aware of your posture while you are at work and when carrying out other daily activities. Practise stretching and strengthening exercises every day to improve the range of motion of all your joints.

INFINITY NECK STRETCHES

⊕ What they do
▸ Keep the cervical (neck) part of the spine flexible and counteract stiffness.
▸ Contribute to a healthy spinal circulation.
▸ Prevent tension from building up in the neck.

⊛ How to do them
1. Sit tall in any comfortable position. Relax your shoulders, arms and hands. Close your eyes or keep them open. Relax your jaw and breathe regularly throughout the exercise.
2. Visualize the Infinity symbol (a figure eight lying on its side). Trace its outline with your nose. Do this slowly and smoothly, 5 or more times.
3. Repeat the exercise in the other direction five or more times. Rest.

⊘ Note
You may also do these neck stretches while standing.

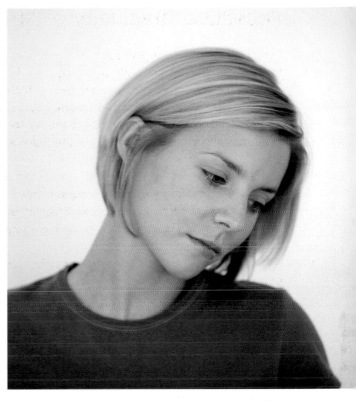

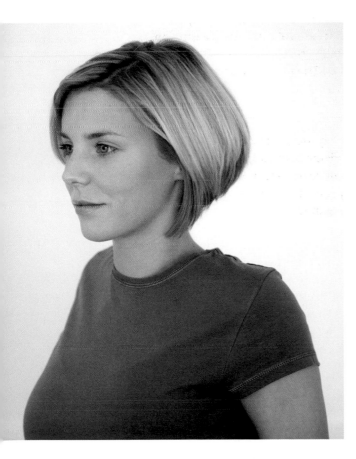

SHOULDER CIRCLES

⊕ What they do
▸ Enhance the effects of the Infinity Neck Stretches.
▸ Keep the shoulder joints moving freely and prevent stiffness.
▸ Improve circulation in the shoulders.
▸ Prevent a build up of tension in the shoulders.

⊛ How to do them
1. Sit tall in any comfortable position. Close your eyes or keep them open. Relax your jaw and breathe regularly throughout the exercise.
2. Draw imaginary circles with your shoulders. Do so slowly and smoothly 5 or more times. Pause briefly.
3. Repeat the shoulder rotations five or more times in the opposite direction

⊘ Note
You may also do the Shoulder Circles while standing.

FIGURE-EIGHT WRIST ROTATIONS

⊕ What they do
▸ Keep hands, wrists and fingers supple.
▸ Improve circulation in these parts and strengthen them.
▸ Prevent tension from building up in the hands.

⊛ How to do them
1. Sit or stand tall in any comfortable position. Relax your jaw and breathe regularly throughout the exercise.
2. Imagine a large figure-eight lying on its side in front of you. Trace its outline with open hands, slowly and smoothly, 5 or more times. Pause briefly.
3. Repeat the exercise in the opposite direction 5 or more times. Rest.

⊘ Notes
You may do it first with one hand and then the other.

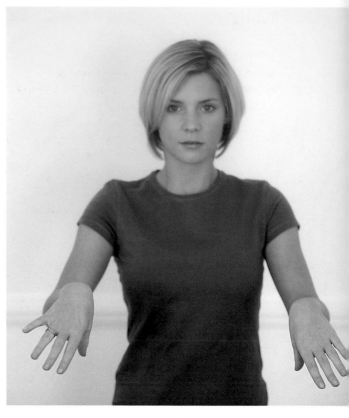

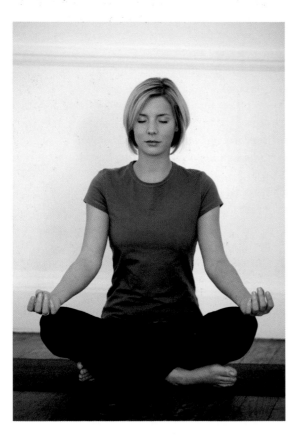

HUMMING BREATH (BHRAMARI PRANAYAMA)

⊕ What it does
▸ Provides a means of release for difficult sensations, such as pain and fatigue, through the vocalization of sound.
▸ Promotes a sense of calm by focusing your awareness on a repeated sound and diverting your attention from disturbing stimuli.

⊛ How to do it
1. Sit tall in any comfortable position. Relax any obviously tense parts. Relax your jaw and breathe regularly. Close your eyes.
2. Inhale through your nose as slowly and as deeply as you can without strain.
3. Exhaling through your nose slowly and steadily, also make a humming sound, like that of a bee. Continue the humming. It should last as long as the exhalation does.
4. Repeat steps 2 and 3 as many times as you wish.

THE CLOCK

⊕ What it does
▸ **Exercises and strengthens eye muscles.**
▸ **Counteracts eyestrain, which can result from long periods of close eye work and glare.**

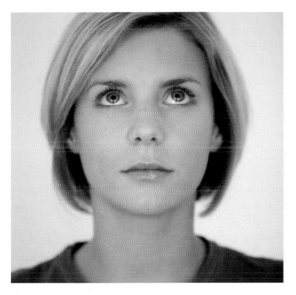

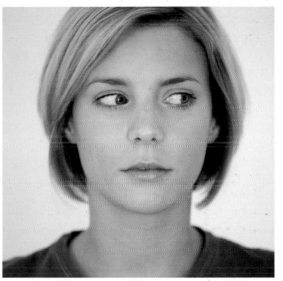

⊛ How to do it

1. Sit tall in any comfortable position. (You may also stand.) Relax your arms and hands. Relax your jaw and breathe regularly throughout the exercise.

2. Imagine looking at a large clock in front of you. Gaze at the number 12 for a second or two, then move your eyes to look at the number 1.

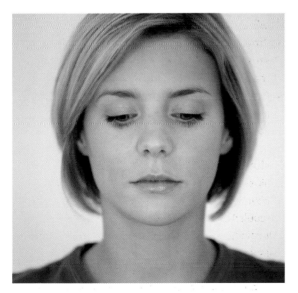

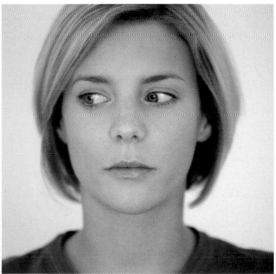

3. Continue shifting your gaze to each consecutive number, going clockwise, until you reach 12 again. Rest briefly.

4. Repeat the exercise, going anti-clockwise.
5. Finish the exercise by blinking several times to moisturize your eyes with natural fluid.

Breathing problems

Breathing difficulties may stem from a variety of disorders, including heart disease; a lung condition such as chronic bronchitis or emphysema; respiratory infections; allergies (page 119) or asthma (page 56). In all these cases, difficult or laboured breathing, which is known as dyspnoea, is often manifest. Dyspnoes can also occur in anxiety (page 78) and after strenuous exercise.

Chronic airflow limitation (CAL)
Also known as chronic obstructive pulmonary disease (COPD) or chronic obstructive lung disease (COLD), this condition refers to a number of disorders that affect the movement of air in and out of the lungs.

With CAL and other chronic lung disorders, airways lose their elasticity and may collapse during exhalation (breathing out), especially when this is forced or laboured. Consequently, air is trapped beyond the point of collapse.

Chronic bronchitis
This is chronic inflammation of the mucous membrane lining the bronchial tubes (passageways leading from the windpipe to the lungs). Symptoms include increased mucus production and cough.

Emphysema
Derived from a Greek word that means "to inflate", emphysema is a chronic lung disease characterized by abnormal distension of the alveoli (air sacs). This stretching of the air sacs is sometimes so great that the walls between them break down. Symptoms include dyspnoea on exertion and a cough that produces mucus.

Hyperventilation
Many of us tend to quicken our breathing in response to stress. Breathing can then sometimes become so rapid that a state of hyperventilation (overbreathing) occurs.

Continued rapid breathing results in an oxygen surplus and a carbon dioxide depletion. It is the carbon dioxide level in the body that determines the control of respiration in the brain.

Should overbreathing be prolonged, the extra oxygen constricts blood vessels and hinders the release of oxygen from haemoglobin in the tissues. (Haemoglobin is the iron-containing pigment of the red blood cells. Its function is to carry oxygen from the lungs to the tissues.) Consequently, less blood will be carrying less oxygen.

Hyperventilation can lead to anxiety which can also develop into panic. The person experiencing either one tends to feel frightened and powerless. Hyperventilation can also precipitate a fall in blood pressure, feelings of lightheadedness, nausea, tingling and numbness of the hands and feet, and muscle spasms.

Breathing retraining

Chronic lung disorders and other respiratory problems can be exhausting and also anxiety provoking. They can leave those experiencing them feeling helpless and sometimes hopeless.

Breathing retraining (respiratory rehabilitation) programmes help those who have such problems to preserve the greatest functional capacity, develop a sense of normality and recapture some of the joy of living through education and physical conditioning. These programmes do so by helping to prevent airflow obstruction, treat breathing complications and improve the overall quality of life.

They also aim to decrease the work and increase the efficiency of breathing, improve oxygenation (the supplying of oxygen) and promote feelings of being in control. In addition, these programmes teach people with respiratory disorders how to relax. Not surprisingly, many of the techniques taught are based on yoga breathing exercises (see Pranayama, pages 8–9).

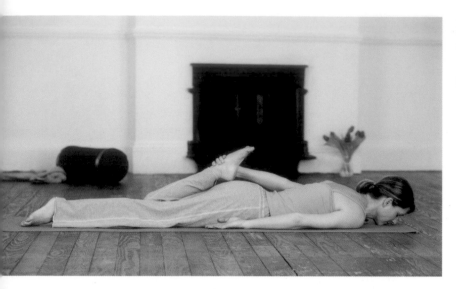

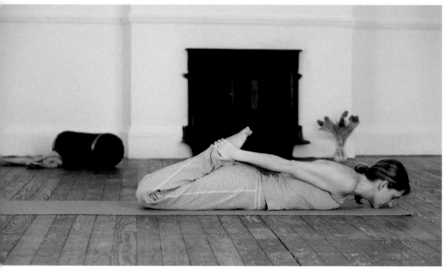

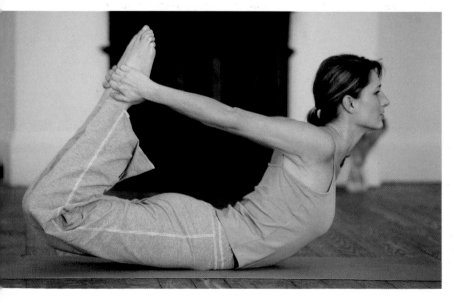

BOW POSTURE (DHANURASANA)

⊕ What it does

▶ Expands the chest to facilitate deep breathing and enhance the delivery of oxygen to the tissues.

▶ Keeps the spine flexible and conditions the back and abdominal muscles.

▶ Improves the functioning of structures in the kidney area (at the small of the back) and in the abdomen.

▶ Helps to relieve constipation.

⊛ How to do it

1. Lie on your abdomen with your chin on the mat and legs stretched out behind you and comfortably separated. Relax your jaw and breathe regularly.
2. Bend one leg and hold the foot, ankle or lower leg with the hand on the same side.
3. Bend the other leg and hold it, as above.
4. Exhale and push your feet away and upwards. This action will raise your legs and arch your torso. Keep your head up.
5. Breathe regularly while holding this posture for three to five seconds to start with; longer as you become more practised.
6. Carefully resume your starting position. Rest.

⊘ Note

A good position in which to relax following the Bow Posture is the Pose of a Child (page 108).

⊙ Caution

Omit this exercise if you have a hernia, a serious heart condition or if you are pregnant.

RHYTHMIC DIAPHRAGMATIC BREATHING

⊕ What it does

▸ Permits a maximum intake of oxygen with minimum effort.

▸ Reduces respiratory rate and consequently heart rate.

▸ Increases tidal volume (the volume of air breathed in and out in one normal breathing cycle, that is, inhalation and exhalation).

▸ Decreases residual volume (the volume of air remaining in the lungs at the end of maximal respiration).

▸ The up-and-down motion of the diaphragm gently massages abdominal organs and so improves their circulation and functioning.

▸ Promotes a natural even flow of breath which strengthens the nervous system and relaxes the body.

▸ Increases exercise tolerance.

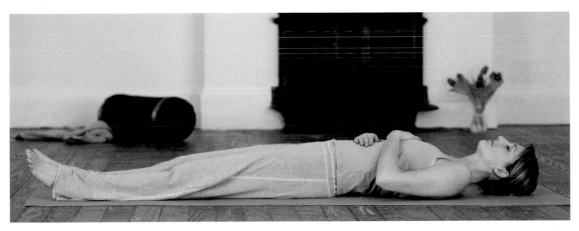

⊛ How to do it

1. Lie on your back with your legs stretched out and your arms at your sides. You may place a cushion, pillow or folded towel under your head. Relax your jaw and breathe regularly. Close your eyes or keep them open.

2. Rest one hand lightly on your abdomen, just beneath your breastbone.

3. Rest your other hand lightly on your chest, just below the nipple.

4. With your abdomen as relaxed as possible, inhale through your nose slowly, smoothly and as fully as you comfortably can. As you do so, the hand on the abdomen will rise as the abdomen moves upwards. There should be little or no movement of the hand on the chest.

5. Exhale through your nose slowly, smoothly and as completely as you can without force. As you do so, the hand on the abdomen will move downwards as the abdominal muscles contract.

6. Repeat steps 4 and 5: inhalation followed by exhalation, several times in smooth succession.

7. Relax your arms and hands. Breathe regularly.

⊘ Notes

• *You may breathe out through pursed lips (page 54).*

• *If you begin to feel lightheaded, immediately resume your usual breathing. (If you were practising this exercise while standing, sit down.)*

• *If uncertain whether your abdomen should rise or fall, think of a balloon: when air is put into it, it expands or grows larger. When air is let out, it deflates or grows flatter.*

• *When you have mastered diaphragmatic breathing while lying down, try it in other positions (sitting upright, reclining or standing). Integrate it into everyday activities such as vacuum cleaning a carpet, walking up and down the stairs or raking leaves in the garden.*

PURSED-LIP BREATHING (WHISPERING BREATH)

⊕ What it does

▶ Allows the airways (leading to the lungs) to remain open longer, thus reducing the amount of air trapped in the air sacs (alveoli). Permits a greater than usual volume of air to be exhaled.

▶ Prolongs exhalation and so promotes a sense of control.

▶ Trains you to control the rate and depth of your breathing and so relieves dyspnoea (difficult breathing) and the anxiety that frequently accompanies it.

⊛ How to do it

1. Sit tall in any comfortable position. Relax your arms and hands. (You may also practise this exercise while lying down or standing.)
2. Relax your jaw and breathe regularly.
3. Inhale through your nose slowly, smoothly and as deeply as you can without strain.
4. Exhale through pursed lips, as if whistling or cooling a hot drink. Do so slowly, smoothly and completely, without force.
5. Repeat steps 2 and 3: inhalation followed by exhalation several times in smooth succession.
6. Close your mouth but do not tighten your jaw, and resume regular breathing.

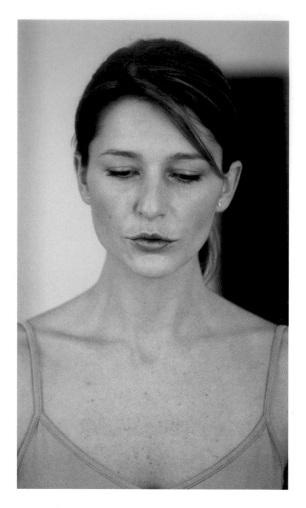

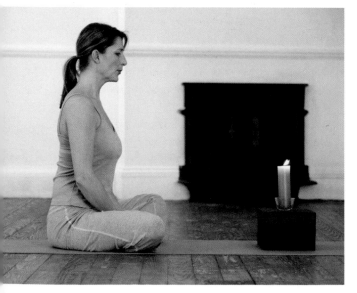

⊘ Notes

• *You may practise this exercise using a lit candle placed on a prop in front of you. Exhale through pursed lips, as instructed above. Blow steadily at the candle flame to make it flicker but not to extinguish it.*

• *When you have mastered the technique, you can dispense with the candle and simply visualize the candle flame.*

• *Be sure to put out the candle at the end of your exercise. Children being taught this technique, using a lit candle, should be supervised.*

• *Integrate Pursed-Lip Breathing into daily activities such as walking up and down the stairs and while waiting at a traffic light.*

SIDEWAYS (LATERAL) STRETCH

⊕ What it does

▸ Facilitates free movement of the ribcage and diaphragm for more efficient breathing.
▸ Keeps the spine flexible.
▸ Tones back and abdominal muscles.
▸ Discourages fat build up at the midriff.

⊛ How to do it

1. Sit tall in any comfortable position. Relax your jaw and breathe regularly.
2. Rest the palm of your right hand on the mat.
3. Inhale and stretch your left arm straight upwards with the palm up.
4. With the lower body kept steady, exhale and stretch your upper torso slowly and smoothly to the right. Relax your wrist or point your fingers to the right.
5. Hold the stretch for five seconds to start with, but keep breathing regularly.
6. Inhale and come upright. Relax your left arm.
7. Repeat, stretching your right arm. Rest.

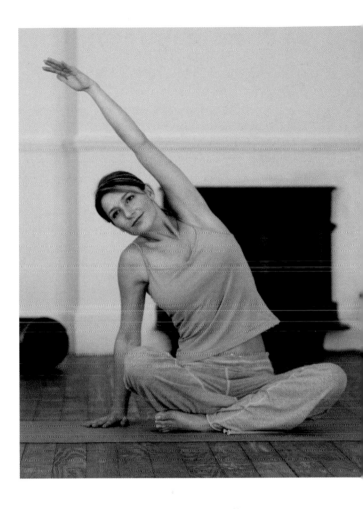

NASAL WASH (NETI)

⊕ What it does

▸ Keeps the nasal passages clear and soothes their mucous lining.
▸ Increases the tolerance of the nasal mucous membrane to irritants.
▸ Promotes physiological harmony by enabling you to breathe freely through the nostrils.

⊛ How to do it

1. Dissolve one-quarter of a teaspoon of salt in a cup of warm water (the approximate concentration of sodium in blood and tissue fluids).
2. Pour a little of the solution into a clean cupped hand. Close one nostril with a thumb or finger and very carefully inhale some of it into the open nostril.
3. Briskly, but not forcefully, breathe out to expel the fluid into a wash-basin or other receptacle.
4. Repeat the procedure with the same nostril once or twice.
5. Repeat the procedure two or three times with the other nostril. Breathe normally and rest.

⊘ Note

Special neti pots are available in stores that sell yoga supplies.

Asthma

Asthma comes from a Greek word that means "panting", and this characterizes what occurs during an asthmatic episode.

In asthma, the muscular tubes through which air flows into and out of the lungs (airways) tighten, become inflamed, swollen and hyperactive, and an excess or mucus is produced. Airflow is thus limited and the result is difficulty in breathing (known as dyspnoea). Other symptoms associated with asthma include wheezing, tightness in the chest, retractions (sucking in of the chest or neck skin), bouts of coughing, fatigue and tingling in the toes and fingers, which indicate hyperventilation (page 50).

Asthma can affect anyone but most frequently appears in young children. Among the agents that can trigger or aggravate an asthmatic episode are cigarette smoke, plant pollens, flowers, grass, animal dander (small scales of dead skin), dust mites, molds, cockroaches, some foods and medicines, cold air and some forms of exercise.

Although infectious agents may trigger an asthmatic episode, asthma is not itself spread by germs and it is not contagious. Emotional stress, although not a direct cause, can undoubtedly provoke or worsen an asthma attack.

Preventing asthma

The best form of asthma prevention is to avoid triggers. The most difficult of these to control is house dust, which is in almost every home, particularly in children's rooms. Try to control the dust build up by removing carpets, curtains and other such dust-collectors; using mattress and pillow covers; improving ventilation; and cleaning regularly.

Asthma and exercise

Although some forms of exercise can bring on an asthmatic episode, suitable exercise should not be avoided by asthma sufferers. Do check with your doctor before engaging in your chosen exercise.

There are many benefits to be derived from regular, appropriate exercise (such as yoga): maintaining the strength and efficiency of the heart and breathing muscles, so that less energy is needed to cope with bothersome symptoms; and building a fit and flexible body, which helps to prevent the excess body weight that can complicate asthma. Exercise also promotes a sense of calm and awareness to enable you to work with your breath and use it to your advantage.

If medication has been prescribed for you, take it before beginning to exercise (check with your doctor) to help prevent asthma symptoms from occurring. Allow 15 to 30 minutes for bronchodilators to activate in your body before you start. (A bronchodilator is a medicine that causes airways to open.)

FISH POSTURE (MATSYASANA)

⊕ What it does

▸ Expands the chest to facilitate deep breathing.
▸ Enhances the functioning of organs in the abdomen and pelvis through the stretching of the mid-trunk and through a gentle internal massage.
▸ Useful in counteracting constipation.

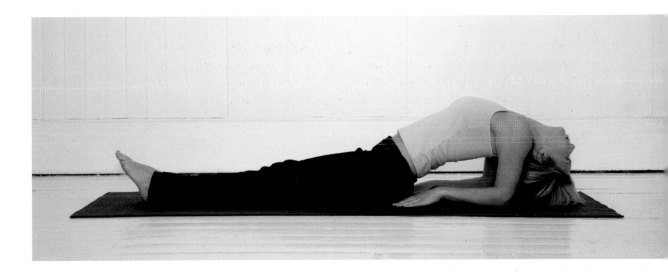

⊛ How to do it

1. Lie on your back with your legs stretched out in front and your arms at your sides. Relax your jaw and breathe regularly.
2. Bend your arms and press on your elbows to help you to raise your chest and arch your back.
3. Very carefully stretch your neck and ease your head towards your shoulders. Gently rest the top of your head on the mat. (Take most of the weight on your bottom and elbows; not on your head.)
4. Hold this posture for a few seconds to start with; longer as you become more comfortable with it. Breathe slowly, smoothly and as deeply as you can without straining.
5. Very carefully ease yourself out of the posture to resume your starting position. Rest.

⊘ Note

The Knee Hug (page 39) is a good posture to do following the Fish.

① Cautions

• *Omit this posture during the first three days of menstruation.*
• *Omit it if you have neck pain or suffer from a balance disorder such as vertigo or dizziness.*
• *If you have a thyroid gland problem, first check with your doctor if you plan to include this posture in your exercise programme.*

DOG STRETCH (ADHO MUKHA)

⊕ **What it does**
▸ Helps to drain mucus that has accumulated in the airways and relieve congestion.
▸ Relieves fatigue in the back and legs.
▸ Helps to maintain the elasticity of the hamstring muscles at the back of the legs. When these muscles shorten, they affect the tilt of the pelvis and so influence posture.

🖐 **How to do it**
1. Start in an all-fours position, on hands and knees. Slope your arms slightly forwards and keep your back level. Relax your jaw and breathe regularly throughout the exercise.
2. Rock forwards slightly, raise your knees and straighten your legs. Straighten your arms. Hang your head down. Aim your heels towards the mat without straining the muscles at the back of your legs.

3. Hold this hips-high, head-low posture for five seconds to begin with; progressively longer as you become more comfortable with it. Keep breathing regularly.
4. Gently rock forwards as you prepare to resume your starting position.
5. Sit on your heels (see Firm Posture, page 20) and rest for a few moments.

✎ **Notes**
• *You may rest in the Pose of a Child (page 108) after doing this exercise.*
• *Note that the Dog Stretch is also part of the Sun Salutation Series (pages 89–91).*

⚠ **Caution**
Do not practise this posture if you suffer from high blood pressure, or have a heart condition or other disorder that produces feelings of lightheadedness or dizziness when you hang your head down.

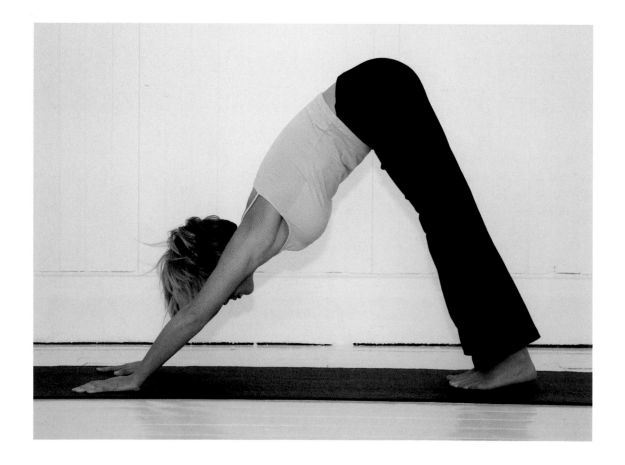

CHEST EXPANDER
(KARMASANA)

⊕ What it does

▸ Facilitates deep breathing.
▸ Counteracts the ill effects that can result from too much bending forwards.
▸ Improves posture.
▸ Reduces tension build up in the shoulders and upper back.

⊛ How to do it

1. Stand tall. Relax your arms at your sides. Relax your jaw and breathe regularly.
2. Inhale and swing your arms behind you. Interlace the fingers of one hand with those of the other. Raise the linked hands as high as you comfortably can without bending forwards.
3. Hold the posture as long as you can without strain, while breathing regularly.
4. Lower your arms and unlock your fingers. Shrug your shoulders a few times before resting.

⊘ Note

You may also practise the Chest Expander in any comfortable seated position.

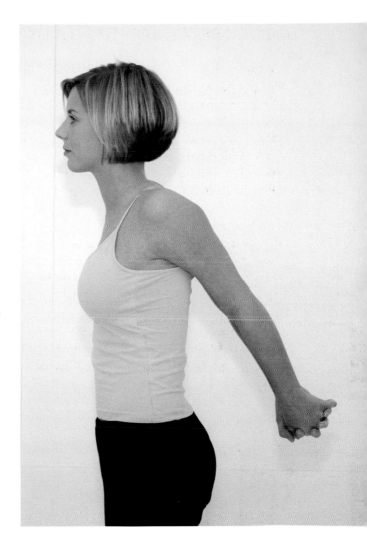

ANTI-ANXIETY BREATH

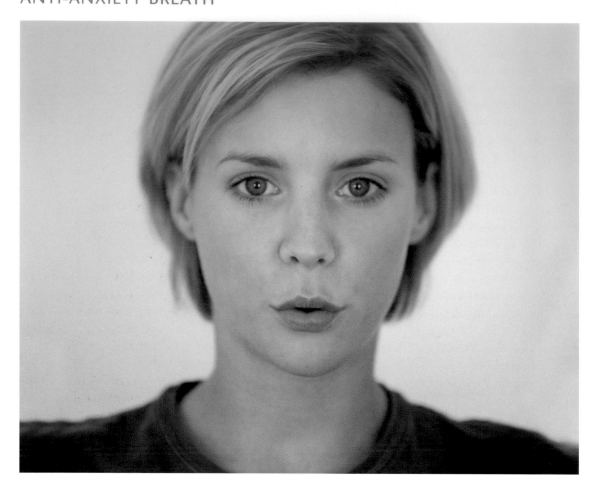

⊕ What it does

▸ **Counteracts anxiety and averts panic.**

▸ **Promotes a sense of being in control.**

▸ **Trains you in prolonging your exhalation, which many people with asthma find difficult to do.**

▸ **Useful in managing disturbing emotions such as anger and frustration.**

⊛ How to do it

1. Sit tall in any comfortable position. Relax your shoulders, arms and hands. Relax your jaw and breathe regularly.

2. Inhale through your nose slowly, smoothly and as deeply as you can without strain.

3. Exhale through your nose (or pursed lips, as if cooling a hot drink) slowly, smoothly and as thoroughly as you can without force.

4. Before inhaling again, do a slow mental count: "one, one thousand", "two, one thousand",

to extend and slow down your exhalation and prevent hyperventilation.

5. Repeat steps 2 to 4, several times in smooth succession, until your breathing has become slower and you begin to feel calm.

6. Resume regular breathing.

⊘ Notes

• *You may also practise this exercise while standing or lying down.*

• *Try combining imagery with breathing. For example, as you inhale, imagine bringing into your system positive and healing qualities such as love, patience, courage and hope. As you exhale, visualize sending away, on the outgoing breath, unhealthy forces such as fear, discouragement and resentment. Use imagery with which you are completely comfortable.*

Blood pressure

Blood pressure refers to the pressure exerted on the walls of arteries and veins and on the chambers of the heart by the heart's pumping action. Blood pressure is given in two readings.

The systolic pressure indicates the contraction of the heart at peak level as it drives blood through the large blood vessels. The diastolic pressure is when the heart is relaxing (dilating) and the blood is at its lowest pressure.

Generally, a normal adult blood pressure reading is considered to be less than 130 (systolic) over less than 85 (diastolic).

Hypertension (high blood pressure)

This is a condition in which an individual has a higher blood pressure than that judged to be normal. The primary factor in hypertension is the narrowing or hardening of the arteries.

High blood pressure is often without symptoms, and millions of people are unaware that they have it until it is revealed during a routine medical examination.

Factors contributing to high blood pressure include: heredity, stress (page 88), being overweight (page 113), smoking, high alcohol intake, substance abuse, high salt intake and the use of certain medicines, including some oral contraceptives. Some women may also suffer hypertension as a result of pre-eclampsia, which is an abnormal condition of pregnancy.

Untreated hypertension can lead to serious illness, such as coronary (heart) artery disease, congestive heart failure, stroke or cardiovascular (heart and blood vessels) disease. As with so many other conditions, prevention is better than cure and sensible measures can help to avoid high blood pressure.

POSE OF TRANQUILLITY (SAVASANA)

⊕ **What it does**

▸ Of all the relaxation techniques, this is probably the one most employed, best loved and most effective. Practised regularly it:

▸ Promotes a state of total and deep relaxation that helps to create a foundation for wellbeing and for healing.

▸ Facilitates coping with stress.

▸ Helps to lower blood pressure to within normal range.

▸ Breaks the fear–tension–pain cycle and so helps with pain control and anxiety.

▸ Has a calming effect on the mind, and also on internal organs and other structures.

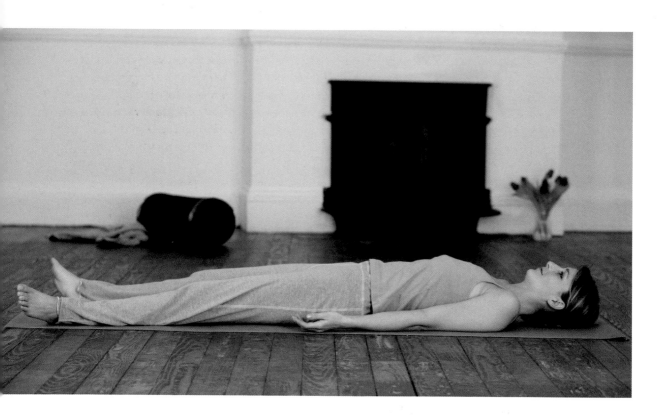

⊛ How to do it

1. Lie on your back with your legs stretched out in front and comfortably separated. Relax your arms a little away from your sides, with your palms up. Rest your head on a small pillow if you wish. Close your eyes, relax your jaw and breathe regularly throughout the exercise.

2. Stiffen your legs, push your heels away and pull your toes towards you. Hold the tightness for a few seconds then completely relax your feet and legs. (Maintaining the muscle contraction, or tightening, is referred to has "hold" and letting go as "relax".)

3. Tighten your buttocks. Hold for a few seconds. Relax.

4. On an exhalation, press the small of your back (waist) towards or against the mat. You will feel your abdomen tighten. Hold for a few seconds while breathing regularly. Relax.

5. Inhale and squeeze your shoulder blades together. Hold. Exhale and relax. Breathe regularly.

6. Exhale and tighten your abdomen. Inhale and relax. Breathe regularly.

7. Take a slow, comfortably deep inward breath and sense your chest expanding. Exhale smoothly and completely. Relax your chest and abdomen. Breathe regularly.

8. Make fists, stiffen and raise your arms off the mat. Hold. Let your arms fall to the mat, relaxed. Relax your hands and fingers.

9. Keeping your arms relaxed, shrug your shoulders. Hold. Relax.

10. Gently roll your head from side to side a few times. Reposition your head.

11. On an exhalation, open your mouth widely, stick out your tongue, open your eyes widely as if staring and tense all your facial muscles.

12. Inhale, close your mouth and eyes and visualize all tension and fatigue draining away.

13. For the next few minutes, or longer if you have time, lie in complete surrender: let the surface on which you are lying take your full weight. With each exhalation, sink more heavily into that surface. With each inhalation, imagine breathing in positive forces such as peace, healing and refreshment.

14. Gently turn your head from side to side a few times, rotate your ankles and leisurely stretch your limbs. Get up safely (page 64).

⊘ Notes

- You may practise the Pose of Tranquillity in other positions (page 64). Modify the exercise instructions accordingly.

- Keep a sweater, light blanket or a pair of warm socks handy. Use them as necessary to prevent you from becoming cold as your body temperature lowers during relaxation.

- Step 11 of the instructions describes a yoga exercise known as the Lion (Simhasana). It may be practised as a separate posture, while sitting or standing, to help to avert a sore throat or prevent it from worsening.

- In step 13 of the instructions, use imagery with which you feel most comfortable. You can, for instance, visualize lying on a warm, sandy beach listening to waves lapping at the shore, and feeling the gentle caress of the breeze on your skin.

- Practise this exercise where you can be assured of 10 to 20 minutes of uninterrupted time.

- When you are familiar with the techniques, you can dispense with alternately tightening and relaxing muscle groups. Instead, give mental suggestion to each part of the body in turn; for example, "Shoulders, let go of your tightness. Relax."

- You may record the exercise instructions on a tape-recorder or ask a friend with a pleasing voice to do so. Speak slowly and soothingly. Listen to the recording as the need arises, such as before going to sleep at night or when feeling anxious.

ALTERNATIVE POSITIONS

If you are unable to practise the Pose of Tranquillity in a supine position, try one of the following:

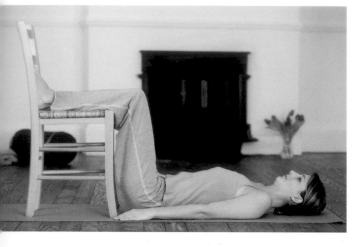

LEGS ON A CHAIR

1. Lie on your back on a non-skid mat on the floor, with a small pillow under your head and neck, if you wish. Relax your arms at your sides. Relax your jaw and breathe regularly.
2. Lifting one leg at a time, bend your legs so that they form a 90-degree angle at the hip and knee joints. Rest your lower legs on a padded chair seat.
3. When ready to get up, carefully lift one leg at a time off the chair seat, roll onto your side and come into a sitting position (see below).

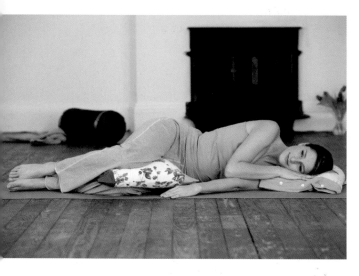

LYING ON YOUR SIDE

Some people find lying on their side more comfortable than lying on their back. Ancient yoga practitioners believed that lying on the right side (Daksinasana) is conducive to sound sleep.

1. Choose a firm surface on which to lie.
2. Lie on your side, with your hip and knee joints bent. Rest your head on a pillow. Also place pillows under and between bony prominences such as the knees and ankles.
3. When ready to get up, do so carefully (see below).

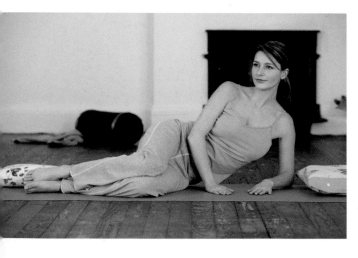

GETTING UP SAFELY FROM LYING

Avoid sitting straight upwards from a supine position. Instead, use the following technique while breathing slowly and smoothly with your jaw relaxed.

1. Roll onto your side, bend your knees and bring them closer to your chest.
2. Use your hands to help push you onto your hip.
3. Carefully pivot yourself until you are sitting evenly on your bottom.
4. Slowly stand up.

CANDLE CONCENTRATION (TRATAK)

⊕ What it does

▸ Traditionally one of six purification exercises, Candle Concentration stimulates certain nerve centres to improve concentration and produce a calming effect.

▸ Useful as a pre-sleep exercise for those who suffer from insomnia.

▸ Strengthens the eyes.

⊛ How to do it

1. Place a lit candle on a prop in front of you so that the flame is at, or just below, eye level.

2. Sit tall in any comfortable position. Relax your shoulders, arms and hands. Relax your jaw and breathe regularly throughout the exercise.

3. Look steadily at the candle flame, for about a minute to start with. Blink if you need to do so.

4. Now close your eyes and try to retain or recall the image of the flame. Do not be anxious if it escapes from you. Open your eyes and try the exercise again.

5. Gradually increase practice time to three or more minutes.

6. Extinguish the candle when you have finished.

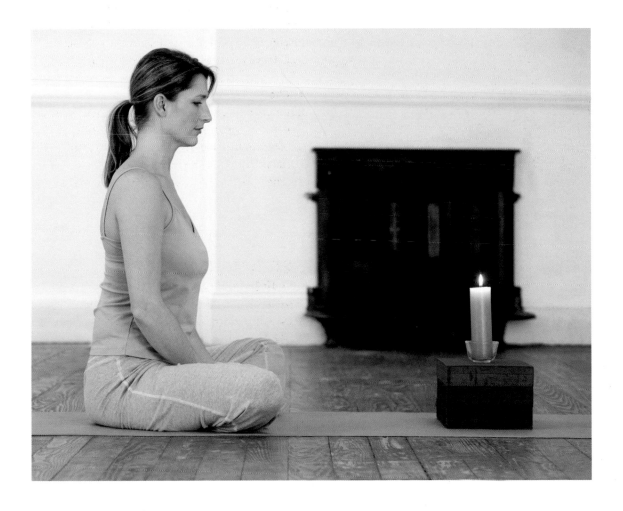

Digestive problems

Digestive disorders are widespread and among the most common reasons why people take medication or see a doctor.

Problems occurring in the stomach and intestines include heartburn and chest pain, abdominal cramps, nausea and vomiting, constipation, diarrhoea, difficulty swallowing, belching, bloating, intestinal gas, indigestion, bleeding, and weight loss.

Heartburn

Heartburn refers to a burning sensation in the chest. It may begin in the upper abdomen and progress to the neck. It may also produce a sour taste in the mouth, especially when you are lying down.

Causes of heartburn include: overeating and being overweight, lying down too soon after eating, having too much alcohol and caffeine, and going to bed at night with a full stomach.

If you experience heartburn frequently, or if you take antacids almost daily, you should consult a doctor: the heartburn may be a symptom of a more serious disorder such as gastroesophageal reflux disease (GERD) or gallstones. Should the heartburn worsen, particularly if it is accompanied by pain radiating to an arm, it may signal a heart attack and you should seek medical help immediately.

Indigestion

Indigestion describes a number of symptoms including: abdominal discomfort, nausea, heartburn, bloating and belching.

Among the causes are stomach inflammation (gastritis), peptic ulcer (ulcer of the stomach and small intestine), food allergy (page 119), and some medicines. Indigestion may also be triggered by intense emotion.

Less commonly, it may be a symptom of a disorder of the pancreas or gallbladder.

Having an occasional bout of indigestion is usually no cause for worry. Should it occur regularly, however, do consult a doctor.

Gas

When you swallow food, you often also swallow air. When air builds up in your digestive tract it can lead to belching or bloating, or to flatulence (excessive gas in the intestine) when the air travels down to the colon. Constipation can also contribute to intestinal gas.

There are some measures you can take to help prevent this build up of gas, for example, limiting the intake of foods that are gas-producing, such as peas, beans, cabbage, bran cereals and fried or other fatty foods, and even some artificial sweeteners. In doing this, however, be careful not to miss out on essential vitamins and minerals. Consulting with a dietitian may be helpful.

Exercise regularly. Regular exercise helps to prevent constipation and reduce gas build up and bloating.

Constipation

The longer the waste products of ingested food stay in your colon, the less water it will contain. This is because the colon absorbs water from food residues. In time, this waste matter will become dry and hard to expel.

With age, muscles of the digestive tract may become less active and more sluggish, and constipation may become a problem. Other causes of constipation include not drinking enough liquids, particularly water; not eating adequate supplies of foods that contain fibre (such as whole grains, vegetables and fruits), and exercising infrequently. Some medicines which slow down digestion can also produce constipation. These include narcotics and antacids containing aluminum.

Although constipation can usually be relieved, it can sometimes point to a more serious problem if it persists. Should you experience the following symptoms, do seek medical advice and help:

- You notice a recent change in bowel pattern for which there is no apparent explanation.
- You've gone for a week or more without a bowel movement, despite taking dietary measures or exercising.
- You've noticed blood in your stools or have had intense abdominal pain.

STICK POSTURE
(YASTIKASANA)

⊕ What it does
▸ Relaxes tense abdominal and pelvic muscles.
▸ Allows for maximum stretching of the body.
▸ Helps to counteract faulty postures.

⊛ How to do it
1. Lie on your back with your legs stretched out in front and your hands at your sides. Relax your jaw and breathe regularly. Close your eyes or keep them open.
2. Inhale slowly, smoothly and as deeply as you comfortably can while stretching your arms and hands straight overhead. At the same time, stretch your legs, push your heels away and bring your toes towards your body.
3. Hold the posture, for five seconds to start with, but keep breathing regularly.
4. Exhale and release the stretch. Bring your arms back beside you. Rest.

⊘ Note
Please turn to page 116 for a standing version of this posture.

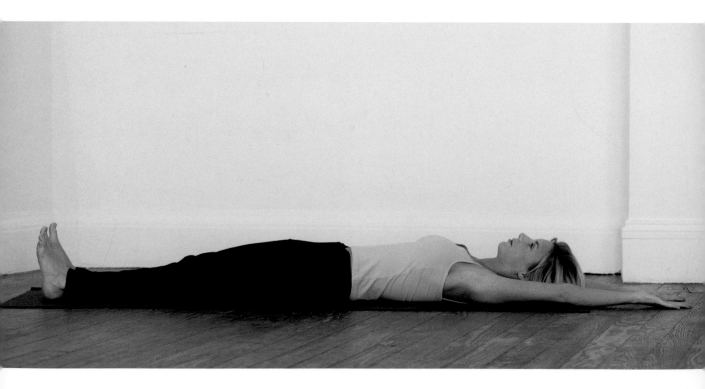

ANGLE BALANCE

⊕ What it does

▸ Strengthens abdominal muscles to provide efficient support for abdominal organs.

▸ Counteracts constipation.

▸ Helps to prevent backache (strong abdominal muscles are necessary for a healthy back).

▸ Keeps you focused, which has a calming effect.

⊛ How to do it

1. Sit with your knees bent and the soles of your feet flat on the mat. Relax your jaw and breathe regularly throughout the exercise.
2. Carefully tilt backwards to lift your feet off the mat.
3. Stretch your arms straight forwards, outside your legs.
4. Slowly and attentively begin to straighten your legs. Adjust your tilt so as to maintain balance.
5. Hold the posture as long as you comfortably can while breathing regularly.
6. Bend your knees and relax your arms to come out of the posture and resume your starting position. Rest.

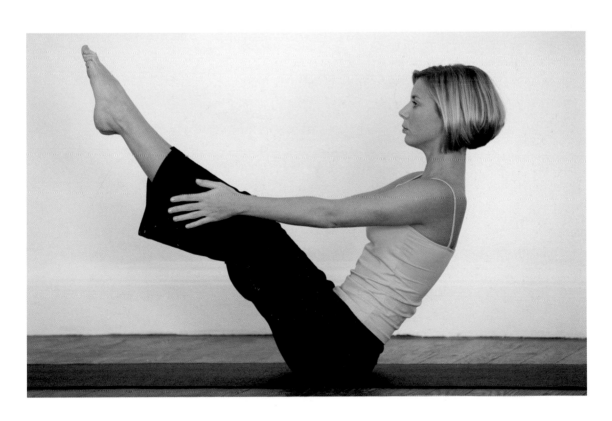

HALF LOCUST (ARDHA SALABHASANA)

⊕ What it does
▸ Gently stimulates abdominal organs and helps to improve their functioning.
▸ Combats constipation.
▸ Strengthens your back and legs.
▸ Enhances the functioning of the adrenal glands and the kidneys through a gentle internal massage.

⊛ How to do it
1. Lie on your abdomen, with your chin on the mat and your legs close together. Keep your arms straight and close to your sides. Relax your jaw and breathe regularly.
2. Exhale and slowly raise one straight leg as high as you comfortably can. Keep your hands flat by your sides.
3. Hold the raised-leg posture as long as you can without strain, while breathing regularly.
4. Slowly lower your leg to the mat, synchronizing the movement with regular breathing.
5. Repeat the exercise with the other leg. Rest.

⊘ Note
The Pose of a Child (page 108) is a good position in which to relax after doing the Half Locust.

ⓘ Caution
Avoid the Half Locust if you have a hernia or a serious heart condition. Omit it from your exercise programme if you are pregnant.

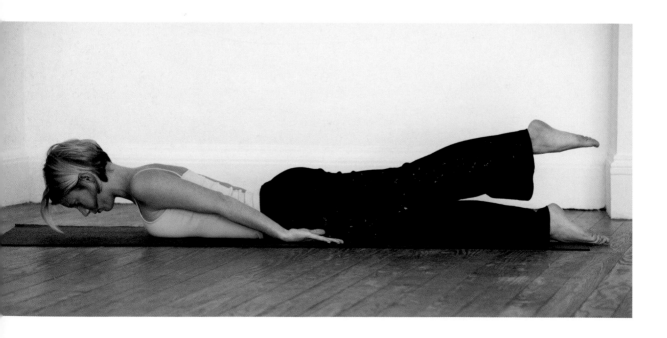

FULL LOCUST (SALABHASANA)

⊕ What it does
▸ The benefits of this exercise are the same as for the Half Locust.

⊛ How to do it
1. Lie on your abdomen with your chin on the mat and your legs close together. Keep your arms straight and close to the sides of your body. Relax your jaw and breathe regularly.
2. On an exhalation, lift both legs together, as a unit, as high as you can with absolute comfort. Keep your arms straight and your palms on the mat.
3. Hold the raised legs posture, for three to five seconds to start with, while breathing regularly.
4. Carefully and with control, lower your legs as a unit to the mat. Rest.

⊘ Note
The Pose of a Child (page 108) Is a good position In which to relax after doing the Full Locust.

① Caution
These are the same as for the Half Locust opposite.

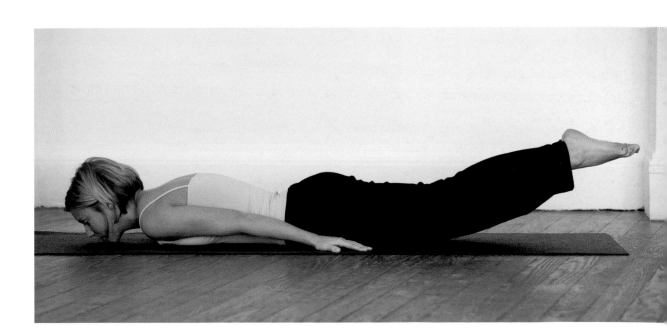

A SIMPLE MEDITATION

⊕ What it does

▸ Diverts your attention from disturbing stimuli and concentrates it on one point of focus. This is wonderfully calming to the nervous and other body systems, and to all internal structures.

▸ See also Meditative Practices (pages 9–10).

⊛ How to do it

1. Sit tall in any comfortable position. Relax your jaw and breathe regularly. Relax your shoulders, arms and hands. Close your eyes.

2. Inhale slowly and smoothly through your nose.

3. While exhaling slowly and smoothly through your nose, mentally say "one".

4. Repeat steps 2 and 3 again and again in smooth succession. If your attention strays, gently guide it back to your breathing and to the repetition of "one" on each exhalation.

5. When ready to end your meditation, do so slowly: open your eyes, leisurely stretch your limbs or gently massage them. Never come out of meditation abruptly.

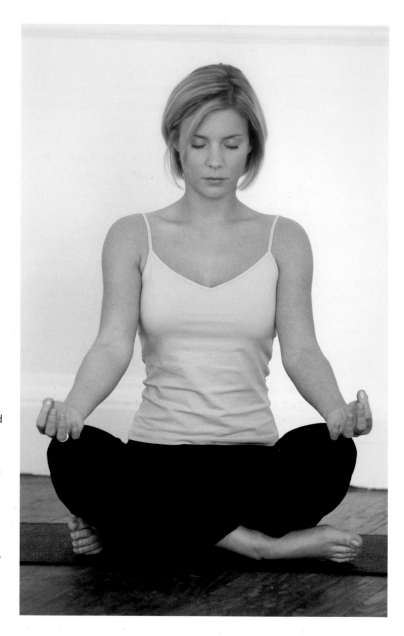

⊘ Notes

• *Do not be disheartened if your attention wanders frequently when first attempting to meditate. In time and with perseverance this will occur less frequently.*

• *Instead of using the word "one", you may choose any alternative word or short phrase. Particularly effective is something related to your belief system, such as "amen", "om", "shalom", "salaam" or "love and peace".*

Urinary Problems

The following are among the most common urinary problems:

Urinary frequency

When urination occurs more often than every two hours, urinary frequency is the term used to describe the condition. Causes include: decreased bladder capacity, changes in urine volume, inflammation and psychological disorders.

Dysuria

Painful or difficult urination is called dysuria. Often described as a burning sensation, dysuria is usually associated with infection and inflammation of the bladder and related structures.

Nocturia

Excessive urination during the night is known as nocturia. Sleep is disturbed by the need to urinate more than twice nightly. Nocturia is associated with those conditions listed above for urinary frequency, and also with some circulatory problems.

Cystitis

This is an inflammation of the bladder. It is usually the result of a urinary tract infection (UTI). It causes frequent and painful urination.

Cystitis and other UTIs are about eight times higher in women than in men, probably because the female urethra (canal for the discharge of urine) is shorter and located closer to the anus and vagina. This makes it easier to become infected.

Self-help measures to relieve cystitis include: avoiding caffeinated and alcoholic beverages, which tend to irritate the bladder lining; and increasing fluid intake, particularly water and cranberry juice (the latter acidifies the urine).

Urinary incontinence

This term describes the inability to retain urine, usually because of a loss of control of the sphincter muscle which opens and closes the urethra. It may result from a disease or from an injury involving the brain or spinal cord. It may also be a side effect of a number of drugs, including tranquillizers, rapid-acting diuretics and blood pressure-lowering agents.

Stress incontinence of urine

This is an involuntary loss of urine, usually when coughing, sneezing or laughing. It occurs when the pressure within the abdomen increases, in a person with weak sphincter muscles.

Urinary incontinence in women is commonly the results of surgical or obstetric trauma, weakened and prolapsed pelvic organs following repeated childbirth, and a decline in oestrogen, as occurs in menopause.

In men, an enlarged prostate gland or weakening genito-urinary structures (of the genitals and urinary organs) following prostate gland surgery may produce urinary stress incontinence.

STAR POSTURE

⊕ What it does

▸ Improves pelvic circulation.
▸ Tones the muscles of the inner thighs and pelvic floor.
▸ Keeps the spine flexible.
▸ Helps to relieve minor backaches.
▸ Keeps the hip, knee and ankle joints moving freely and prevents stiffness.

⊛ How to do it

1. Sit tall on your mat, with your legs stretched out in front of you. Relax your jaw and breathe regularly.
2. Fold one leg inwards and rest the foot beside the other knee.
3. Fold the other leg and put the soles of the feet together. Maintain this distance between feet and body. Clasp your hands around your feet.
4. On an exhalation, slowly and smoothly bend forwards, at your hip joints rather than at your waist, bringing your face as close to your feet as you comfortably can. Relax your neck.
5. Hold the posture as long as you can, without strain, while breathing regularly.
6. Slowly come back to an upright sitting position, synchronizing movement with regular breathing.
7. Relax your arms and hands and rest.

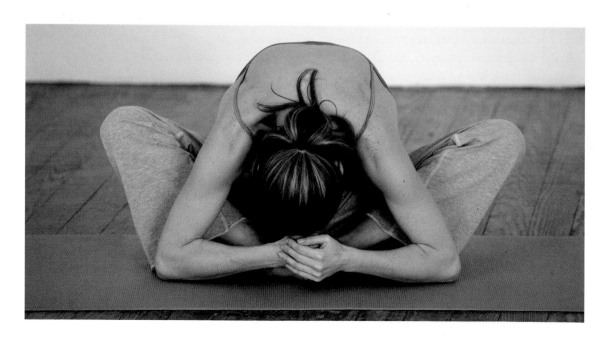

BUTTERFLY

⊕ What it does

▸ Helps to keep the ankle, knee and hip joints moving freely and prevents stiffness.

▸ Stretches and tones the muscles of the inner thighs and groin.

▸ Improves circulation in the structures of the lower pelvis.

⊛ How to do it

1. Sit tall on your mat, with your legs stretched out in front. Relax your jaw and breathe regularly throughout the exercise.

2. Fold one leg inwards. Fold in the other leg and bring the soles of your feet together. Clasp your hands around the feet and bring them comfortably close to your body.

3. Rhythmically and at a moderate pace, alternately lower and raise your knees, like a butterfly flapping its wings. Do this from 10 to 20 times.

4. Carefully unfold your legs and stretch them out, one at a time. Rest.

ⓘ Caution

Omit this exercise if you have pain in your pubic area.

▽ Variation

1. Sit on your mat. Rest your palms on the mat beside your hips.

2. Fold your legs inwards, one at a time, and bring the soles of the feet together.

3. Alternately lower and raise your knees, from 10 to 20 times, in smooth succession.

4. Stretch out your legs. Relax your arms and hands and rest.

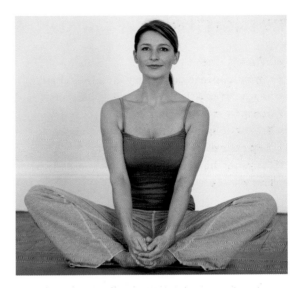

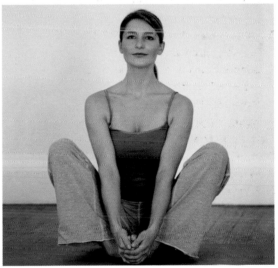

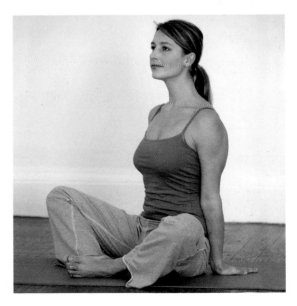

TRIANGLE POSTURE (TRIKONASANA)

⊕ What it does

▸ Conditions many ordinarily underexercised muscles of the torso and legs.

▸ Tones the muscles of the abdomen, to provide better support for organs and other structures in the abdomen and pelvis.

▸ Tones the muscles of the back.

▸ Stretches and strengthens the leg muscles, which affect pelvic tilt and therefore posture.

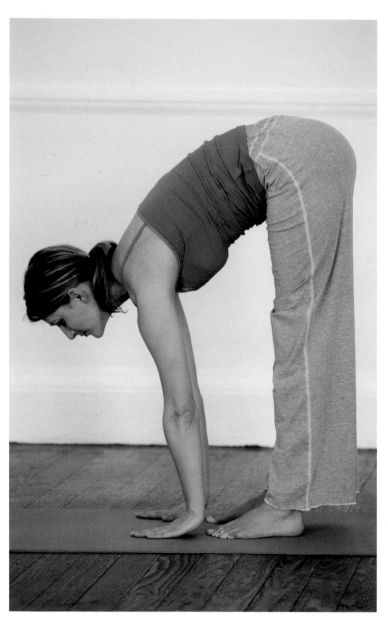

⊛ How to do it

1. Stand tall with your feet together and arms at your sides. Relax your jaw and breathe regularly.

2. Exhale and, keeping your upper torso straight, bend forwards at the hip joints and try to touch the mat in front of you. Keep your legs straight and your head up. (If unable to touch the mat, simply bend forwards as far as you comfortably can, with arms stretched ahead of you.)

3. Hold the posture as long as you can, without strain, while breathing regularly.

4. Inhale and come upwards very carefully, to resume your starting position. Rest.

PELVIC FLOOR EXERCISE

Apart from the respiratory diaphragm, there is also a pelvic diaphragm, which is a sling-like muscular support for the pelvic organs. It is located between the legs and extends from the coccyx or "tailbone" (at the base of the back) to the pubic bone.

The structure of the pelvic diaphragm, or pelvic floor, combined with the forces of gravity and frequent increases in pressure within the body, make it vulnerable to sagging, somewhat like a hammock.

Studies have shown that when pelvic floor muscles are paralyzed, the respiratory diaphragm descends and the volume of air remaining in the lungs at the end of maximal respiration (residual volume) increases. The pelvic diaphragm thus has more of a supporting role than is generally realized. In fact, it plays a significant part in respiration, since it markedly affects residual volume.

The exercises that are the most effective in strengthening and re-educating weakened pelvic floor muscles involve not only these muscles, but also those of the back and abdomen and the respiratory diaphragm as well, since they all work together as a unit.

⊛ How to do it

1. Sit, stand or lie down comfortably. Make a quick top-to-toe mental check of your body and relax any obviously tense parts. Relax your jaw and facial muscles and breathe regularly.
2. Inhale slowly, smoothly and as deeply as you comfortably can through your nose. Note the rising of your abdomen as you do so.
3. Through your nose, or pursed lips as if cooling a hot drink, exhale gradually and as completely as you can without force while at the same time tightening the pelvic floor muscles (at the lowest point of your torso, between your coccyx at the back and your pubic area at the front). Note the contraction of your abdomen as you exhale.
4. Inhale slowly and steadily while relaxing your pelvic floor muscles.
5. Repeat steps 3 and 4, one or more times: steady exhalation along with tightening your pelvic floor muscles, followed by a relaxing of the muscles as you inhale. Rest afterwards.
6. You may repeat the exercise later in the day.

⊛ Variation

1. Try combining visualization with this exercise. For example, imagine being in a lift (elevator), going from the ground floor to perhaps the fourth or fifth floor of a building. On an exhalation, begin to tighten your pelvic floor muscles, a little at a time, to correspond with your ascent to each floor. Let the muscle tightening build up to the maximum as you reach the top floor.
2. When your exhalation and muscle contraction are complete, inhale and relax your pelvic floor muscles by degrees as you descend to the ground floor.
3. Repeat the exercise one or more times before resting and breathing regularly.
4. You may repeat the exercise later in the day.

Anxiety

The word "anxiety" comes from the Latin verb "angere" which means to press tightly or choke. Indeed, those who have experienced anxiety report symptoms of pressure and other similar unpleasant sensations.

Anxiety is perhaps best described as a generalized feeling of apprehension or dread, and also of uncertainty and powerlessness. People who have suffered from anxiety are often unable to pinpoint the source of their unease or predict when the dreaded event, whatever it may be, will occur. Fear of some identifiable danger, however, can also produce anxiety.

Theories about the origins of anxiety include that it: stems from past unconscious conflict, beginning in infancy or childhood; is a learned behaviour; is a result of biochemical imbalances in the central nervous system (CNS). Usually at the root of anxiety, however, is a combination of physical and environmental factors, rather than a single cause.

Anxiety is a normal response. It helps to prepare us for dealing with a perceived threat, and as such it has protective value. In fact, the ability to be anxious may be necessary for survival.

Because anxiety is a response to a perceived threat, the body mobilizes various forces to meet the challenge, so as to prepare us for "fight or flight". Manifestations of this include accelerated heart rate, palpitations, a feeling of pressure in the chest, rapid breathing, nausea, heartburn, diarrhoea, shakiness, restlessness, sleeplessness, frequency of urination, sweating, hot and cold spells, increased muscle tension, rapid speech, lack of coordination, hypervigilance, poor concentration, forgetfulness, errors in judgement, impatience and diminished productivity.

Stress of any kind can precipitate or worsen feelings of anxiety. Examples include a forthcoming exam, or interview, or a life-changing event such as marriage. Since individual perceptions differ, however, what may be dismissed by one person as inconsequential may prove to be distressing for another.

Anxiety may be triggered or aggravated by certain substances including caffeine, alcohol and some drugs used to treat erectile dysfunction.

Anxiety disorder

When feelings of anxiety persist and become excessively intense, and when they significantly impair functioning, an anxiety disorder may be suspected.

Anxiety disorders are categorized as: generalized anxiety disorders, phobias (including social phobia and agoraphobia), panic and panic disorders, obsessive compulsive disorder and post-traumatic stress disorder.

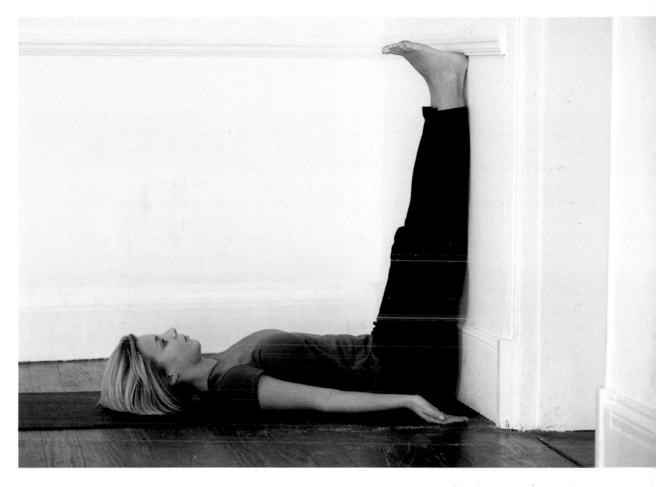

LEGS UP (VIPARITA KARANI)

⊕ What it does

▶ **Soothes the nervous system. Promotes harmony and deep relaxation of body and mind.**

⊛ How to do it

1. Lie near a wall. Relax your jaw and breathe regularly.
2. Bend your legs and carefully manoeuvre your body so that by raising your legs you can rest your feet, one at a time, against the wall.
3. Ease your bottom as close to the wall as you comfortably can so that, ideally, your legs are straight up and form a 90-degree angle with your torso. Relax your arms a little away from your sides. Close your eyes.
4. As you inhale slowly, smoothly and as deeply as you comfortably can, imagine bringing into your system peace, refreshment and healing, or any other positive qualities you desire.
5. As you exhale slowly, smoothly and as thoroughly as you can without strain, visualize banishing from your system tension, anxiety and fatigue or any other negative qualities you wish to be rid of. Use your exhalation to let your body sink more deeply into the surface upon which you are lying.
6. Repeat steps 4 and 5 again and again in smooth succession.
7. When you are ready to get up do so slowly and carefully: bend your legs, ease them back onto the floor and get up safely (page 64).

⊙ Caution

Omit this posture if you have recently formed blood clots in your veins. Check with your doctor.

PURSED-LIP BREATHING (WHISPERING BREATH)

⊕ What it does

▸ Permits a greater than usual volume of air to be exhaled and so facilitates deep inhalation.

▸ Prolongs exhalation and so promotes a sense of control.

▸ Trains you to control the rate and depth of your breathing and so relieves dyspnoea (difficult breathing) and the anxiety that often generates it.

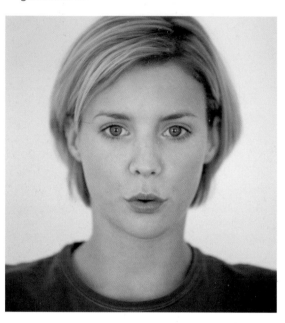

⊛ How to do it

1. Sit tall in any comfortable position. Relax your arms and hands. (You may also practise this exercise while lying down or standing.) Relax your jaw and breathe regularly.
2. Inhale through your nose slowly, smoothly and as deeply as you can without strain.
3. Exhale through pursed lips, as if whistling or cooling a hot drink. Do so slowly, smoothly and completely, without force.
4. Repeat steps 2 and 3: inhalation followed by exhalation several times in smooth succession.
5. Close your mouth, but do not tighten your jaw, and resume regular breathing.

⊘ Notes

• *You may practise this exercise using a lit candle placed on a prop in front of you, at or just below eye level. Exhale through pursed lips, as instructed above. Blow steadily at the candle flame to make it flicker but not to extinguish it.*

• *When you have mastered the technique, you can dispense with the candle and simply visualize the candle flame.*

• *Be sure to put out the candle at the end of your exercise. Children being taught this technique, using a lit candle should be supervised.*

• *Integrate Pursed-Lip Breathing into daily activities such as walking up and down the stairs and while waiting at a traffic light.*

ANTI-ANXIETY BREATH

⊕ What it does

▸ Counteracts anxiety and averts panic.

▸ Promotes a sense of being in control.

▸ Trains you in prolonging your exhalation and so counteracts the rapid breathing that can lead to hyperventilation.

▸ Useful in managing disturbing emotions.

⊛ How to do it

1. Sit tall in any comfortable position. Relax your shoulders, arms and hands. Relax your jaw and breathe regularly.
2. Inhale through your nose slowly, smoothly and as deeply as you can without strain.
3. Exhale through your nose (or pursed lips, as if cooling a hot drink) slowly, smoothly and as thoroughly as you can without force.
4. Before inhaling again, do a slow mental count: "one, one thousand", "two, one thousand", to extend and slow down your exhalation and prevent hyperventilation.
5. Repeat steps 2 to 4, several times until your breathing has slowed and you begin to feel calm.
6. Resume regular breathing.

⊘ Notes

• *You may also practise this exercise while standing or lying down.*

• *Try combining imagery with breathing.*

ALTERNATE NOSTRIL BREATHING (NADI SHODHANAM)

⊕ What it does

▸ There is, in health, a predictable alternating of breath flow between the right and left nostrils. For about two hours, breathing is predominantly through one nostril and then it shifts to the other. This is a natural biological rhythm.

▸ A persisting blockage of one nostril for more than a few hours can be a sign of impending ill health. Such a state can be precipitated by various occurrences, including: emotional upsets, sleep disturbances, nutritional deficits and infection.

▸ By deliberately changing the flow of air from one nostril to the other in a regular fashion, Alternate Nostril Breathing helps to maintain or to restore the body's natural biological rhythm. It is a soothing exercise that helps to counteract anxiety. It is also an antidote for sleeplessness.

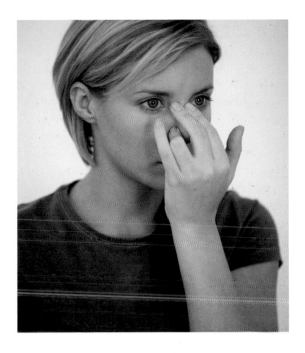

⊛ How to do it

1. Sit tall in any comfortable position. Relax your jaw and breathe regularly.
2. Rest one hand in your lap, on your knee or on the armrest of your chair.
3. With your other hand raised in front of you, arrange the fingers as follows: fold the two middle fingers towards the palm (or rest them lightly on the bridge of the nose once the exercise is in progress). Use your thumb to close off one nostril, and your ring finger (or ring and little fingers) to close off the other, as necessary.
4. Close your eyes and begin. Close your left nostril and inhale slowly, smoothly and as deeply as you comfortably can through your right nostril.
5. Close your right nostril, releasing closure of the left and exhale slowly, smoothly and completely through your left nostril.
6. Inhale through your left nostril.
7. Close your left nostril, releasing closure of the right. Exhale. This completes one round of Alternate Nostril breathing.

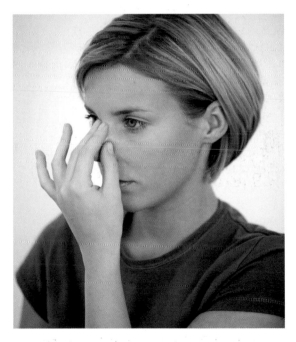

8. Repeat the entire sequence (steps 4 to 7) several times in smooth succession. You may try three to five rounds to start with and increase the number of rounds as you become more familiar with the exercise.
9. Relax your right arm and hand. Rest and breathe regularly.

Depression

Most of us have probably experienced brief episodes of sadness, dejection or discouragement. A major depressive episode, however, is generally characterized by at least five of the following symptoms (including the first two listed) almost continuously for at least two weeks:

• Depressed mood, loss of interest or pleasure, weight loss or gain, sleep disturbance (page 110) such as sleeplessness or sleeping too much, increased or decreased physical activity, fatigue or loss of energy (page 106), feelings of worthlessness, impaired concentration and thoughts of death or suicide.

Among the stressors that can precipitate depression are a bereavement or the loss of something significant to us; a combination of life-changing events in a relatively short period (such as a new job, a change in residence and getting married); physiological changes (such as a serious illness or the adverse effects of certain drugs).

Conventional treatments for depression include medicines (such as antidepressants), psychotherapy ("talk therapy") and cognitive behavioural therapy. The latter attempts to help change distorted perceptions and thought patterns so as to help you view the world and yourself more realistically. In selected cases, ECT (electroconvulsive therapy) is employed. This procedure involves the induction of a brief convulsion (seizure) by passing an electric current through the brain. It is used mostly in cases where patients are not responding to drug and other therapy.

Post-partum depression

This form of depression can occur from two weeks to 12 months after a woman has given birth. Usually, however, it appears within six months of delivery. It is seen in 10 to 15 percent of women. It is marked by mood swings and often heralds a bipolar disorder (known as "manic depression"). There is a 50 percent chance of recurrence with the next pregnancy.

Post-partum blues

These are brief episodes of mood swings and tearfulness that occur within one to five days after giving birth. They are experienced by up to 80 percent of women.

HALF SHOULDERSTAND (ARDHA SARVANGASANA)

⊕ What it does

▸ Enhances the blood supply to nervous structures within the head.

▸ Counteracts the downward pull of gravity by relieving congestion in the body's lower structures.

▸ Tones the muscles of the neck, back and abdomen.

▸ Revitalizes the organs within the trunk and enhances the circulation and functioning of the lymphatic, nervous and endocrine systems (including the thyroid gland, which is sometimes linked to depression)

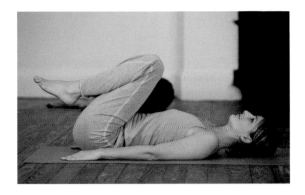

⊛ How to do it

1. Lie on your back with your legs stretched out in front and your arms at your sides. Relax your jaw and breathe regularly throughout the exercise.
2. Bring one bent knee then the other to your chest.
3. Straighten and raise one leg at a time to point your feet upwards.
4. Exhale and kick backwards with both feet at once to bring your hips off the mat. Support your hips with your hands.
5. Maintain this posture for as long as you are absolutely comfortable in it, while breathing regularly.
6. To come out of the posture, rest your hands on the mat, close to your body. Keep your head pressed to the mat and very slowly lower your torso, starting with you upper back, onto the mat.
7. Bend your knees and stretch out your legs one at a time. Rest.

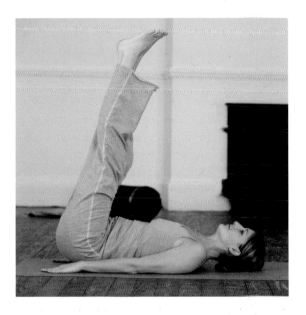

ⓘ Caution

Do not practise this posture during your menstrual period. Omit it from your exercise programme if you have an ear or eye disorder, high blood pressure, heart disease or other cardiovascular disorder. Check with your doctor.

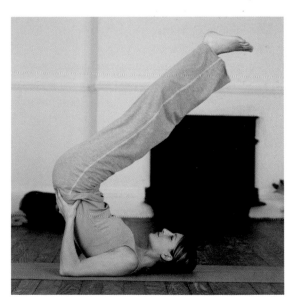

FULL SHOULDERSTAND (SARVANGASANA)

⊕ What it does

▸ The benefits derived from the Full Shoulderstand are the same as for the Half Shoulderstand. In addition, the Full Shoulderstand, through the contraction of muscles at the front of the neck, combined with gentle pressure of chin on chest, has a regulating effect on the thyroid gland. (An underactive thyroid gland is sometimes linked to depression. The gland can also become overactive, and symptoms of this can be sweating, shaking and anxiety.)

⊛ How to do it

1. Lie on your back with your legs stretched out in front and your arms at your sides. Relax your jaw and breathe regularly.
2. Bring one bent knee then the other to your chest.
3. Straighten and raise one leg at a time to point your feet upwards.
4. Exhale and kick backwards with both feet at once to bring your hips off the mat. Support your hips with your hands.
5. Gradually move one hand at a time towards your upper back until your body is vertical. Your chin should be in contact with your chest.
6. Hold the posture for as long as you are comfortable while breathing regularly.
7. To come out of the posture, tilt your legs slightly backwards. Rest your arms on the mat beside your torso. Keep your head pressed to the mat and slowly lower your body, starting with your upper back, to the mat. Bend your knees, stretch out your legs one at a time and rest.

ⓘ Caution

These are the same as for the Half Shoulderstand. In addition, omit the Full Shoulderstand if you suffer from neck pain.

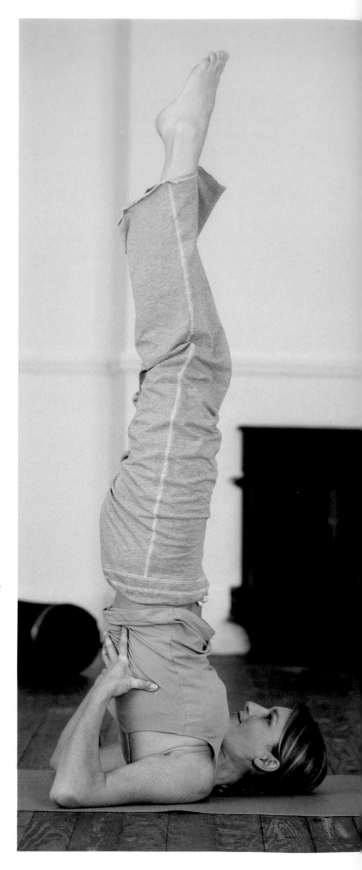

PLOUGH POSTURE
(HALASANA)

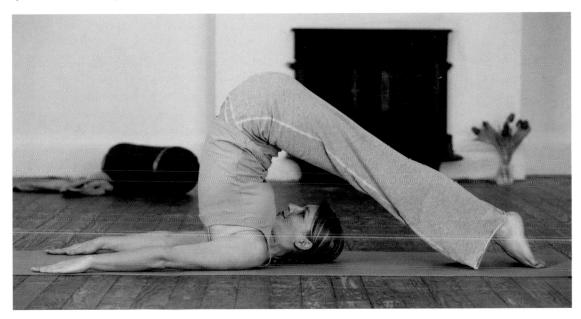

⊕ What it does

▸ The Plough Posture exerts gentle traction on the spinal column. This enlarges the vertebral foramina (openings through which spinal nerves pass) and so eases pressure on these nerves. It also enhances circulation in the spinal cord, and improves the functioning of internal organs supplied by these nerves.

⊛ How to do it

1. Lie on your back with your legs stretched out in front and your arms at your sides, palms turned down. Relax your jaw and breathe regularly.
2. Bring one knee then the other to your chest.
3. Straighten and raise one leg at a time and point your feet upwards.
4. Exhale and kick backwards with both feet at once to bring your hips off the mat. Keep your legs straight and together if you can.
5. Push your feet towards the mat behind your head. Do not let your hips move past your shoulders as this may strain your neck.
6. When you have reached your comfortable limit, hold the posture for five seconds to begin with; increasingly longer as you become more practised in the technique.

7. To resume your starting position, slowly, smoothly and carefully roll your spine back onto the mat, from top to bottom. Bend your knees and stretch out your legs one at a time. Rest.

⊘ Note

It your feet cannot immediately touch the mat behind you, do not be discouraged. Pile up some cushions behind you, on which to rest your toes. As you become more flexible, you can start removing the cushions until, eventually, you can dispense with them entirely.

⊙ Cautions

- *Do not practise the Plough Posture during the first few days of your menstrual period. Omit it from your exercise programme if you suffer from neck pain, have a spinal disc problem, hernia or uterine prolapse or if you have been diagnosed with osteoporosis (pages 40–41).*
- *Do not let your hips go beyond your shoulders, as this may strain your neck.*

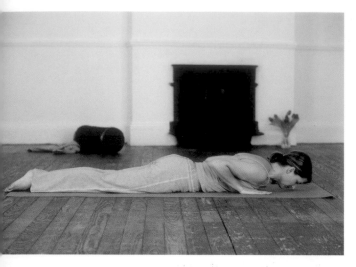

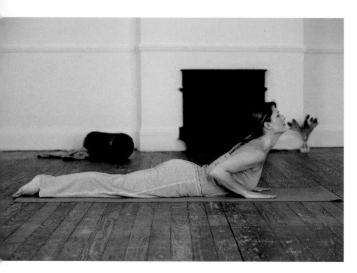

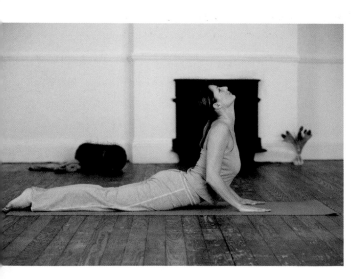

COBRA (BHUJANGASANA)

⊕ What it does

▶ Relieves pressure on nerves branching off the spine.
▶ Enhances spinal circulation.
▶ Helps to keep the spine flexible.
▶ Tones the muscles of the back and abdomen.
▶ Keeps the joints of the shoulders, elbows and wrists moving freely and prevents stiffness.
▶ A good counter-posture to do following the Plough (page 85).

⊛ How to do it

1. Lie on your abdomen, with your head turned to the side and your arms relaxed beside you. Relax your jaw and breathe regularly.
2. Turn your head to the centre and bend your arms at the elbow so that you are face down with your palms resting on the mat, directly beneath your shoulders. Keep your arms close to your sides.
3. Inhale and start slowly arching your back, first touching the mat with your nose and then your chin as you arch your neck; raise your chest and upper abdomen. Do not lift your pelvis.
4. When you have reached your comfortable limit, hold the posture for about five seconds. Keep breathing regularly.
5. Come out of the posture very slowly, lowering your abdomen, chest, chin, nose and forehead to the mat. Synchronize the movement with regular breathing.
6. Relax your arms beside your body and turn your head to the side. Rest.

⊘ Note

The Cobra is also part of the Sun Salutation Series (pages 89–91).

! Caution

Do not practise the Cobra during pregnancy. Omit it from your exercise programme if you have a hernia.

DYNAMIC CLEANSING BREATH (KAPALABHATI PRANAYAMA)

⊕ What it does
▸ Revitalizes the nervous system.
▸ Invigorates the body; counteracts lethargy and fatigue.
▸ Strengthens the abdominal muscles and the diaphragm.
▸ Gives a therapeutic massage to abdominal organs.
▸ Cleanses respiratory passages.

🏃 How to do it
1. Sit or stand comfortably. Relax your shoulders, arms and hands. Relax your jaw and breathe regularly.
2. Inhale slowly, smoothly and as deeply as you can without strain.
3. Exhale briskly through your nose as if sneezing, focusing your attention on your abdomen which will tighten and flatten.
4. Inhalation will occur naturally as you relax your abdomen and chest.
5. Repeat steps 3 and 4 again and again, at a moderate to rapid pace. Start with about six repetitions and gradually increase the number as you become versed in the technique.
6. Resume regular breathing.

⊘ Note
Whereas hyperventilation (page 50) is involuntary, the Dynamic Cleansing Breath is done consciously and with your control. Moreover, it results in a thorough exhalation and a full, spontaneous inhalation. In hyperventilation, by contrast, exhalation is incomplete and there is a sort of desperation to take the next breath. Consequently, carbon dioxide stores are quickly depleted and unpleasant symptoms may appear, such as feelings of lightheadedness and sometimes tingling of hands and feet.

ⓘ Caution
Do not practise this breathing exercise if you have high blood pressure or a heart disorder, epilepsy, a hernia, an ear or eye problem or a herniated ("slipped") disc. Do not practise it during menstruation or if you are pregnant.

Stress

With more demands and expectations in almost every area of life, stress is affecting increasing numbers of people. Stress occurs when the demands of your environment greatly tax or overwhelm your resources for coping with them.

When something happens which is perceived as a threat, the body's sympathetic nervous system is aroused and a number of changes take place. These include an increase in muscle tension (such as rigid neck muscles and a tight jaw), faster heart rate and elevated blood pressure, impaired digestion, shortened blood-clotting time, withdrawal of minerals from bones and a retention of an abnormal amount of salt.

Any event, circumstance or other agent causing or leading to stress is called a stressor. Notable stressors include anxiety, fear, guilt, regret, frustration, anger, resentment and uncertainty. Experienced frequently and allowed to continue unrelieved, these mental states can undermine health by compromising the immune system.

Coping with stress

The single most important key to help you to cope with stress is to try to maintain the highest possible standard of health. There are several key ways to achieve this:

- Eating healthily can increase your resistance to stress by providing essential nutrients that promote stamina.

- Exercising regularly helps to improve mental functioning, decreasing the chances of depression and increasing physical endurance.

- Relaxation (page 10) elicits a parasympathetic nervous system response which is calming. Relaxation is essential for the repair and healing of the physiological consequences of stress.

SUN SALUTATION SERIES (SURYA NAMASKAR)

⊕ What they do

▸ Reduce tension build up and promote relaxation of the whole body.

▸ Facilitate deep breathing.

▸ Tone the muscles of the arms, legs and torso.

▸ Improve circulation.

▸ Improve flexibility and stamina.

▸ Discourage fat build up.

⊛ How to do them

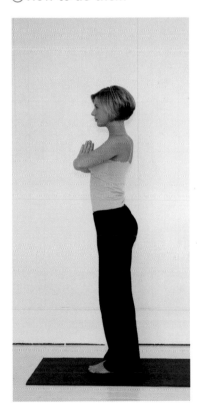
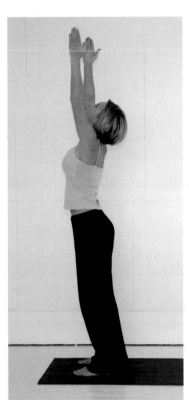
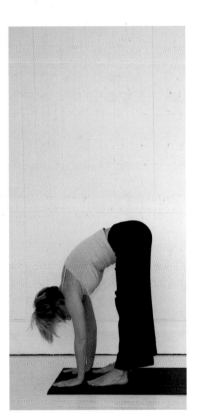

1. Stand tall with your palms touching one another and held in front of your chest, as if in prayer. (This symbolic gesture is a traditional form of paying respect in Indian culture and is known as "namaste".) Relax your jaw and breathe regularly.

2. Inhale, stretch your arms overhead, tighten your buttock muscles and carefully bend slightly backwards without straining.

3. Exhale and carefully bend forwards, at the hip joints rather than at the waist. Rest your hands on the mat outside the feet, if you can.

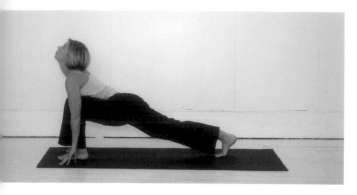

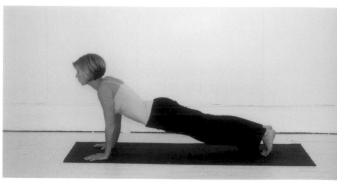

4. Inhale and step back with your right foot, with your toes pointing forwards. Look up.

5. Step backwards with your left foot. Your body weight is now borne by your hands and feet, and your body should be level from head to heels.

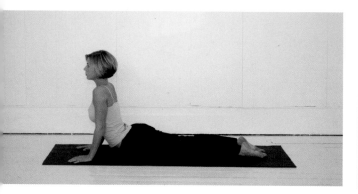

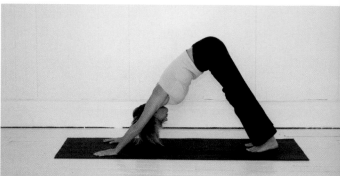

6. Exhale and lower your knees, chin or forehead and also your chest to the mat. Relax your feet with your toes pointing backwards. (This is the "knee-chest" position.)

7. Inhale, lower your body to the mat and slowly and smoothly arch your back, but keep your hips on the mat. Look up. This is the Cobra position (page 86).

8. Exhale, point your toes forwards and press into the mat with your hands to help you raise your hips. Straighten your arms and hang your head down. Aim your heels towards the mat but do not strain your leg muscles. This is the Dog Stretch (page 58).

9. Inhale, look up and rock forwards onto your toes. Step between your hands with your right foot.

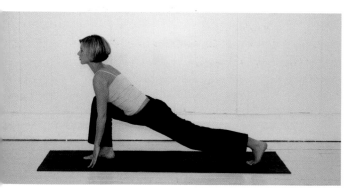

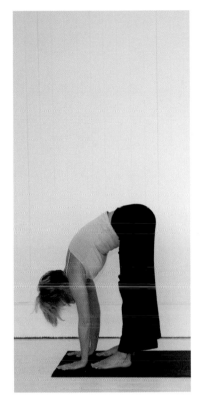
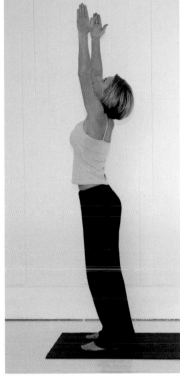
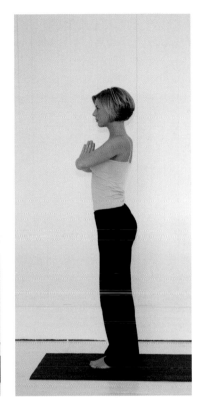

10. Exhale, step between your hands with your left foot and with both feet together, bend forwards slowly and carefully.

11. Inhale and come up slowly and carefully into a standing position, then move smoothly into a backward-bending position with your arms overhead. Tighten your buttock muscles to protect your back from strain.

12. Exhale and resume your starting position, with palms together in front of your chest.

13. Rest briefly and breathe regularly.

⊘ Notes

- *You may perform this Series of 12 movements once to begin with. Gradually increase the number of repetitions as you progress in your practice. With each repetition, alternate the foot that first steps backwards and later comes forwards (steps 4 and 9).*
- *Use the Sun Salutation series as a basis for your own "mini workout". Add a sideward-bending posture such as the Half Moon (page 117), a twisting posture such as the Spinal Twist (page 96) and a balancing posture such as the Tree (page 42) or the Angle Balance (page 69).*
- *Use this series as a warm up before your main exercise programme. To cool down after exercising, do the movements as slowly as possible.*

⚠ Cautions

- *Omit these exercises from your programme if you have varicose veins, venous blood clots or a hernia. Check with your doctor.*
- *See also the cautions for the Cobra (page 86) and the Dog Stretch (page 58).*

POSE OF TRANQUILLITY (SAVASANA) MODIFIED

Here is a modified version of the Pose of Tranquility, described in detail on pages 62–63. The benefits are the same.

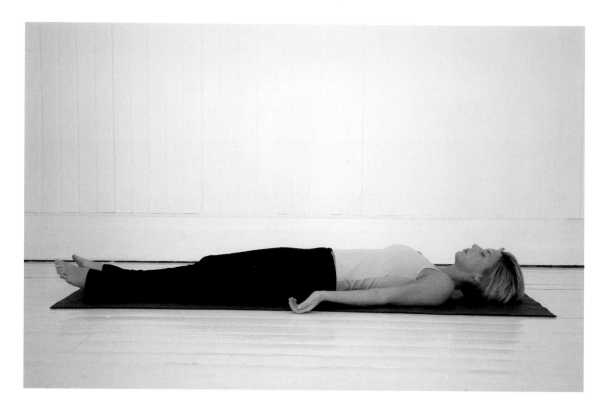

⊛ How to do it

1. Lie comfortably on your back. Relax your jaw and breathe regularly. Close your eyes.

2. Starting with your feet and moving upwards, focus your attention on one part of your body, or group of muscles, at a time and give the gentle prompt to "let go of tightness; release tension; relax completely."

3. A suggested sequence is feet, lower legs, knees, thighs, hips, lower back, upper back, abdomen, chest, hands, forearms, upper arms, shoulders and facial muscles. Spend a few seconds on each area before moving to the next.

4. When you have covered every part, spend a few moments contemplating the soothing rhythm of your breathing which, as you become increasingly relaxed, will be slower and more even.

5. You can spend some extra time using imagery to further enhance your relaxtion. For example, picture yourself in a garden where the flowers are bathing you with their delightful fragrances. You can smell their essences. You can feel your tensions and concerns dissolving or floating away. You surrender yourself to the healing properties of these wonderful blooms. As your relaxation deepens, you sense that you are less troubled, less stressed and more at peace with yourself and with the world.

6. When you are ready to end your meditation, do so in a leisurely fashion and make sure you get up safely (page 64).

VICTORIOUS BREATH (UJJAYI PRANAYAMA)

⊕ What it does
▸ Soothes body and mind.
▸ Counteracts difficult feelings such as irritation and frustration.
▸ Helps to reduce wear and tear on the system.
▸ Replenishes energy.

⊛ How to do it
1. Sit, stand or lie down in any comfortable position, with your spine in good alignment and supported if necessary. Relax your jaw and keep your lips closed but not compressed.
2. Imagine that you are blowing onto a looking glass or window pane, trying to make it foggy, by whispering the syllable "haa".
3. Inhale slowly and smoothly through your nose while pretending to say "haa".
4. Exhale slowly and steadily through your nose while pretending to say "haa".
5. Repeat steps 3 and 4 again and again in smooth succession. You should eventually hear an even, gentle sound which indicates a state of calm.
6. When you are ready to end the exercise, resume regular unvoiced breathing.

⊘ Notes
- *Try integrating this breathing exercise into the Sun Salutation Series (pages 89–91) and into any of the other yoga exercises in your personal programme.*
- *Try incorporating it into activities such as mopping the floor, vacuum-cleaning the carpet, raking leaves or walking up and downstairs.*

The Menopause

The permanent cessation of menstrual activity is known as menopause. The average age for the menopause to begin is 45–55 years. Although menstruation may stop suddenly, it usually takes around five years for menstrual activity to stop altogether. As the production of cyclic hormones (such as oestrogen and progesterone) declines, ovulation and menstruation become less frequent and eventually stop.

Menopause may be induced at any age by the surgical removal of the ovaries, removal of a growth with chemicals (ablation), or radiation of the pelvic organs.

Menopausal symptoms

Common menopausal symptoms include hot flashes, which are sudden involuntary waves of heat that begin in the upper chest and progress to the face and head; hot flushes, which are measurable changes in skin temperature, a visible pink to bright-red change in the skin and perspiration; night sweats, which are hot flashes that occur at night, accompanied by perspiration that can be profuse, and often chills.

Other side effects of the menopause are low energy and fatigue (page 106), mood swings, sleep disturbances (page 110), heart palpitations, dizziness, vaginal irritation, urinary disturbances (page 73) and digestive disturbances (page 66). In addition, there may be some manifestations of osteoporosis (page 40) such as backache and joint pain. Many of these symptoms have been associated with a decline in oestrogen production.

There are a variety of treatments available – both conventional and complementary – to help alleviate the symptoms of the menopause.

PELVIC STRETCH (SUPTA VAJRASANA)

⊕ What it does
▸ Gives a therapeutic stretch to the upper thighs, groin and front of the torso; improves circulation.
▸ Tones the muscles of the back and abdomen.

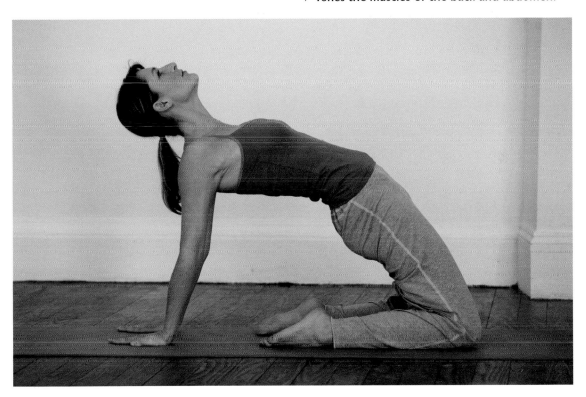

⊛ How to do it
1. Sit on your heels in the Firm Posture (page 20). Relax your jaw and breathe regularly.
2. Rest your hands, with fingers pointing backwards, on the mat behind your feet.
3. On an inhalation, carefully tilt your head back; press on your palms and raise your bottom off your heels.
4. When you have reached your comfortable limit, hold the posture for three to five seconds to start with, longer as you become more practised. Keep breathing regularly.
5. Slowly ease yourself back to sitting on your heels. Rest your hands on your thighs and relax. You may also rest in the Pose of a Child (page 108).

SPINAL TWIST
(MATSYENDRASANA)

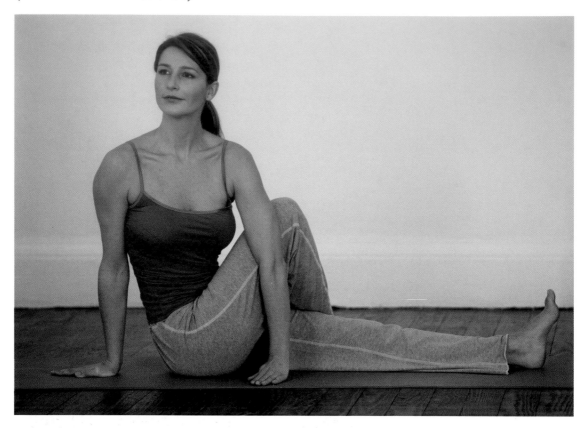

⊕ What it does

▸ Allows maximum torsion (twisting) of the spine to both sides, and so provides a therapeutic massage to nerves branching off the spinal column.

▸ Keeps the spine flexible.

▸ Tones the lower back muscles.

▸ Tones the transverse and oblique abdominal muscles.

▸ Enhances the circulation in the area of the kidneys, at the small of the back.

▸ Revitalizes the adrenal glands, situated on top of the kidneys. (Almost all body systems are influenced by adrenal gland hormones.)

▸ Aids digestion and combats constipation.

⧂ How to do it

1. Sit tall with your legs stretched out in front of you. Relax your jaw and breathe regularly.

2. Bend your right leg over the left one. Place your right foot flat on the mat near your left knee.

3. Exhale and rotate your upper body to the right, as far as you can with absolute comfort. Rest one or both hands on the mat at your right side. Turn your head and look over your right shoulder.

4. Hold the posture as long as you comfortably can while breathing regularly.

5. Slowly and smoothly untwist and resume your starting position. Rest briefly.

6. Repeat the spinal twist on the other side. Relax your arms and legs afterwards.

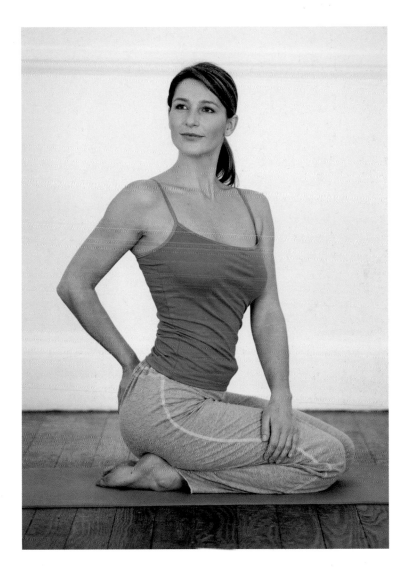

▼ Variation

1. Sit on your heels in the Firm Posture (page 20).
2. On an exhalation, carefully rotate your upper body to the right.
3. Reach across your body with your left hand and hold on to the outside of your right thigh.
4. Rest your right hand on the mat beside you for support, or bend your right arm and place the back of the hand against your lower back. Look over your right shoulder.
5. Hold the posture as long as you comfortably can while breathing regularly.
6. Slowly untwist and resume your starting position. Rest briefly.
7. Repeat the spinal twist on the other side. Relax your arms and legs afterwards.

COOLING BREATH
(SITALI PRANAYAMA)

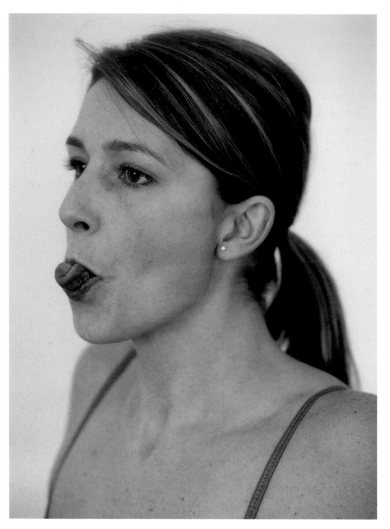

⊕ What it does

▸ Helps to cool an overheated body: when you are angry, when the weather is hot, when you have a fever or when experiencing a hot flash or a hot flush.

▸ Can help to counteract certain cravings, such as for tobacco.

⊛ How to do it

1. Sit tall in any comfortable position. (You can also practise the exercise while standing.) Relax your jaw and breathe regularly.
2. Inhale slowly and smoothly through your nose.
3. Exhale and stick out your tongue; curl it lengthways to form a tube.
4. Inhale slowly and smoothly through this tube.
5. Relax your tongue, pull it in and close your mouth. Breathe regularly.
6. Repeat the exercise (steps 3 to 5) a few times.
7. Resume normal breathing as you rest.

PELVIC FLOOR EXERCISE

The pelvic diaphragm

Apart from the respiratory diaphragm (see page 53), there is also a pelvic diaphragm, which is a sling-like muscular support for the pelvic organs. It is located between the legs and extends from the coccyx ("tailbone") at the base of the back to the pubic bone.

The structure of the pelvic diaphragm, or pelvic floor, combined with the forces of gravity and frequent increases in pressure within the body, makes it vulnerable to sagging, somewhat like a hammock.

Studies have shown that when pelvic floor muscles are paralyzed, the respiratory diaphragm descends and the volume of air remaining in the lungs at the end of maximal respiration (residual volume) increases. The pelvic diaphragm thus has more of a supporting role than is generally realized. In fact, it plays a significant part in respiration, since it markedly affects residual volume.

Consequently, the exercises that are the most effective in strengthening and re-educating weakened pelvic floor muscles involve not only these muscles, but also those of the back, abdomen and the respiratory diaphragm as well, since they all work together as a unit.

⊛ How to do the exercise

1. Sit, stand or lie down comfortably. Make a quick top-to-toe mental check of your body and relax any obviously tense parts. Relax your jaw and facial muscles and breathe regularly.
2. Inhale slowly, smoothly and as deeply as you comfortably can through your nose. Note the rising of your abdomen as you do so.
3. Through your nose, or pursed lips as if cooling a hot drink, exhale gradually and as completely as you can without force while tightening the pelvic floor muscles (at the lowest point of your torso, between your coccyx at the back and your pubic area at the front. Note the contraction of your abdomen as you exhale.
4. Inhale slowly and steadily while relaxing your pelvic floor muscles.
5. Repeat steps 3 and 4, one or more times: steady exhalation along with tightening your pelvic floor muscles, followed by a relaxing of the muscles as you inhale. Rest afterwards.
6. You may repeat the exercise later in the day.

⊛ Variation

1. Try combining visualization with this exercise. For example, imagine being in a lift (elevator), going from the ground floor to perhaps the fourth or fifth floor of a building. On an exhalation, begin to tighten your pelvic floor muscles, a little at a time, to correspond with your ascent to each floor. Let the muscle tightening build up to the maximum as you reach the top floor.
2. When your exhalation and muscle contraction are complete, inhale and relax your pelvic floor muscles by degrees as you descend to the ground floor.
3. Repeat the exercise one or more times before resting and breathing regularly.
4. You may repeat the exercise later in the day.

Menstrual Problems

There are various disorders relating to the menstrual cycle:

Amenorrhoea

This is the absence of menstrual flow when it should normally occur. Amenorrhoea is normal before sexual maturity, after menopause and during pregnancy. Otherwise, it may be due to a disorder of any of the endocrine glands (such as the pituitary), surgical removal of the uterus or ovaries, or the taking of certain medicines. It can also sometimes occur in women with very lean bodies who exercise excessively, or in anorexia nervosa (an eating disorder) when weight loss is extreme.

Bleeding between periods (metrorrhagia)

This is not uncommon and may occur following sexual intercourse. It can also be the result of variations in your usual hormonal cycles, by a change in contraceptive pills or by stress. However, abnormal bleeding may be an early warning sign of cancer, so do see your doctor for a prompt evaluation.

Dysmenorrhoea

Painful menstrual periods, or dysmenorrhoea, is a common condition, occurring (at least occasionally) in almost all women. Although its cause in most cases is not fully understood, it can be due to pelvic disease such as endometriosis, uterine fibroids or pelvic inflammatory disease.

Symptoms accompanying menstrual pain can include backache, headache, nausea and vomiting.

Irregular menstrual periods

These may be due to changes in hormonal levels, to stress or to a drastic change in weight.

Menorrhagia

This is excessive bleeding during menstruation, either in the number of days a period lasts or in the amount of blood lost, or both. If the condition becomes chronic, a woman may suffer anaemia ("iron-poor blood"). Menorrhagia may be caused by uterine fibroids, endocrine gland disorders or pelvic infection.

Premenstrual syndrome (PMS)

This term refers to symptoms that occur several days before menstruation begins. Once the menstrual period starts, the sypmtoms usually subside or disappear altogether. Symptoms characteristic of PMS include fluid retention, bloating, weight gain, breast soreness or pain, fatigue, nausea, vomiting, mood swings, irritability, anxiety, food cravings and difficulty in concentrating.

PELVIC TILT

⊕ What it does

▶ Strengthens the lower back.

▶ Strengthens the abdominal muscles.

▶ Keeps the spine flexible.

▶ Relieves spinal stiffness and minor backaches.

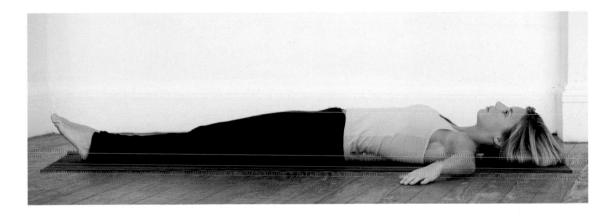

⊛ How to do it

1. Lie on your back with your legs stretched out in front. Relax your arms at your sides. Relax your jaw and breathe regularly.

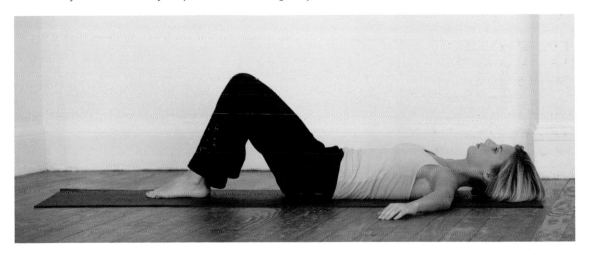

2. Bend your legs and rest the soles of your feet flat on the mat, a comfortable distance from your bottom.

3. Exhale and press the small of your back (waist) towards or against the mat, to decrease the lumbar spinal arch.

4. Hold this downward pressure and the resulting pelvic tilt for several seconds but keep breathing regularly.

5. Inhale and release the pressure. Breathe regularly and relax.

6. Repeat the exercise one or more times if you wish.

7. Stretch out your legs and rest.

PELVIC TILT STANDING

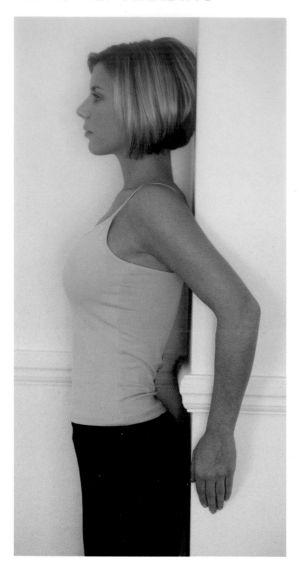 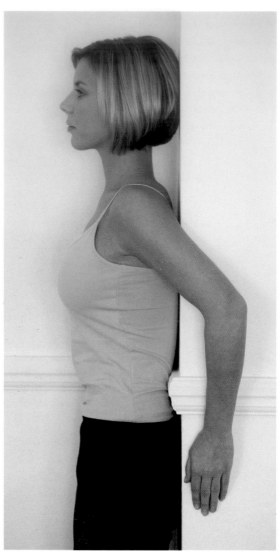

⊛ How to do it

1. Stand tall near a stable prop, such as a wall, post or tree trunk.
2. Exhale and press your lower back towards or against the prop.
3. Hold the pressure for a few seconds while breathing regularly.
4. Inhale and release the pressure. Rest.
5. Repeat the exercise if you wish.

PELVIC TILT SITTING

⊛ How to do it

1. While sitting tall on a firm chair, exhale and press your lower back towards or against the chair back.
2. Hold the pressure for a few seconds while breathing regularly.
3. Inhale and release the pressure. Rest.
4. Repeat the exercise if you wish.

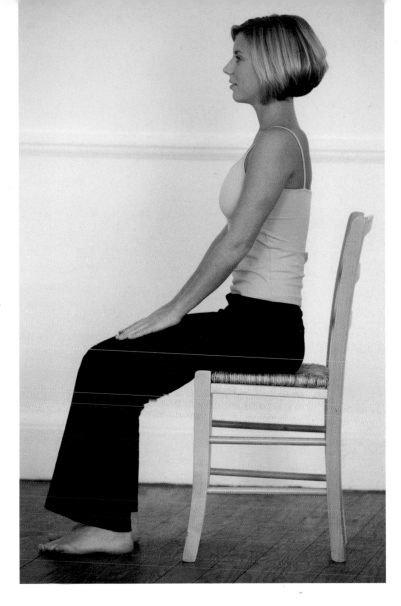

PELVIC TILT ON ALL FOURS

⊛ How to do it

1. Start on all fours on hands and knees, with your back level.
2. Exhale and tuck your bottom downwards. (Your back will become rounded. Focus on moving your hips rather than your shoulders.)
3. Hold for a few seconds while breathing regularly.
4. Inhale and relax your back. Rest briefly.
5. Repeat the exercise several times. See also the Cat Stretch (page 111), steps 1 and 2.

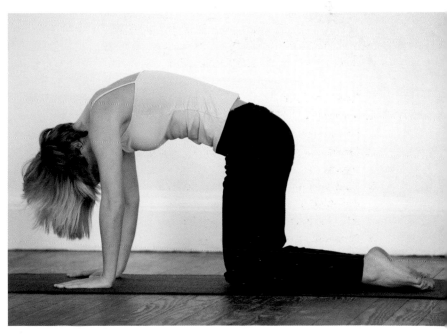

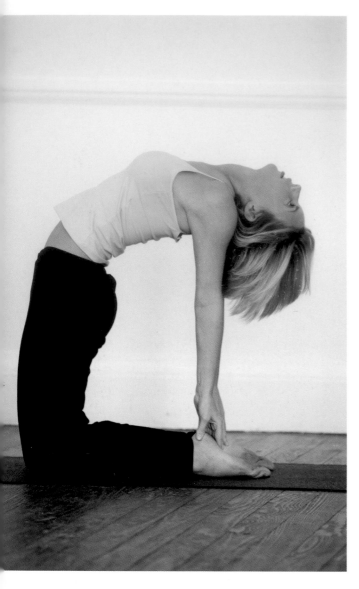

THE CAMEL (USTRASANA)

⊕ What it does

▸ Gently stimulates endocrine glands such as the ovaries, thyroid and adrenals to enhance their functioning.

▸ Has a therapeutic effect on reproductive and urinary organs.

▸ Helps to prevent fat buildup at the midriff.

▸ Expands the ribcage and so facilitates deep breathing.

▸ Strengthens the back and keeps the spine flexible.

▸ Gives a beneficial stretch to the groin and thigh muscles.

⊛ How to do it

1. Kneel down with your legs slightly separated and your toes pointing backwards. Relax your jaw and breathe regularly.
2. Carefully lean backwards so as to rest your right hand on your right heel and your left hand on your left heel.
3. Very carefully tilt your head backwards.
4. Lift your torso and arch your back; keep your hips high.
5. Hold this posture for as long as you can with absolute comfort while breathing regularly.
6. Slowly and carefully resume your starting position by first bringing your head up, followed by your torso. Relax your arms and hands.
7. Sit on your heels and rest, or relax in the Pose of a Child (page 108).

⚠ Caution

Do not practise this posture if you suffer from neck pain or have a spinal disc problem or a hernia.

BUTTERFLY

⊕ What it does

▸ Helps to keep the ankle, knee and hip joints moving freely and prevents stiffness.

▸ Stretches and tones the muscles of the inner thighs and groin.

▸ Improves circulation in the structures of the lower pelvis.

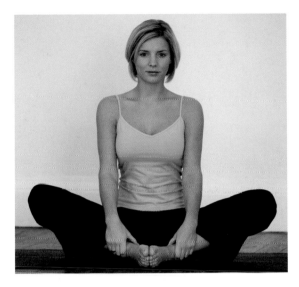

⊛ How to do it

1. Sit tall on your mat, with your legs stretched out in front. Relax your jaw and breathe regularly throughout the exercise.

2. Fold one leg inwards. Fold in the other leg and bring the soles of your feet together. Clasp your hands around the feet and bring them comfortably close to your body.

3. Rhythmically and at a moderate pace, alternately lower and raise your knees, like a butterfly flapping its wings. Do this from 10 to 20 times.

4. Carefully unfold your legs and stretch them out, one at a time. Rest.

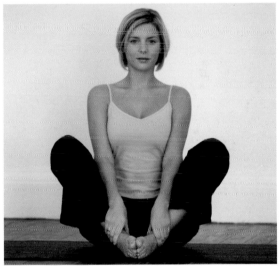

⊘ Caution

Omit this exercise if you have pain in your pubic area.

▽ Variation

1. Sit on your mat. Rest your palms on the mat beside your hips.

2. Fold your legs inwards, one at a time, and bring the soles of the feet together.

3. Alternately lower and raise your knees, from 10 to 20 times, in smooth succession.

4. Stretch out your legs and rest. Relax your arms and hands.

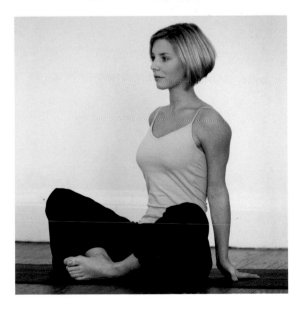

Fatigue

Fatigue is a state in which an individual continually feels exhausted. This usually affects every aspect of life, particlarly one's capacity for physical and mental work, and it can be the first indication of illness.

Chronic fatigue is usually of slow onset, persists over time and is generally not significantly relieved by usual restorative measures. It is also exceedingly debilitating.

The following are characteristic of fatigue: low energy, an increase in the number of physical difficulties experienced, irritability, impaired concentration, loss of interest in one's surroundings, decreased sex drive and proneness to accident.

Fatigue has been associated with: sleep disturbances (page 110), acquired immunodeficiency syndrome (AIDS), thyroid and other endocrine gland disorders, multiple sclerosis (MS), cancer and hepatitis. Fatigue is also commonly seen in depression (page 82), anxiety (page 78) and stress (page 88). It may, in addition, be due to inadequate nutrition.

Chronic Fatigue Syndrome (CFS)

Also known as myalgic encephalomyelitis (ME), CFS is diagnosed where a person has suffered intense fatigue lasting for at least six months and causing at least a 50 percent reduction in one's usual physical activities. The fatigue is also accompanied by some of the following symptoms: sleep disturbances (page 110), muscle weakness, muscle and joint pain, sore throat, painful lymph glands, headache, impaired memory and concentration, and mood swings.

Although the exact cause or causes of CFS are not known, research has focused on the role of enteroviruses, a group of viruses that originally included the polio virus and others that infected the gastrointestinal tract.

CFS can affect anyone at any age, but it is most commonly seen in young and middle-aged women.

CROCODILE (MAKARASANA)

⊕ What it does

▸ Facilitates diaphragmatic breathing and so gives maximum oxygen intake with minimum effort.

▸ Induces deep mental and physical relaxation.

▸ Practised post-natally, it helps the uterus return to its normal position, and tones and flattens the abdomen.

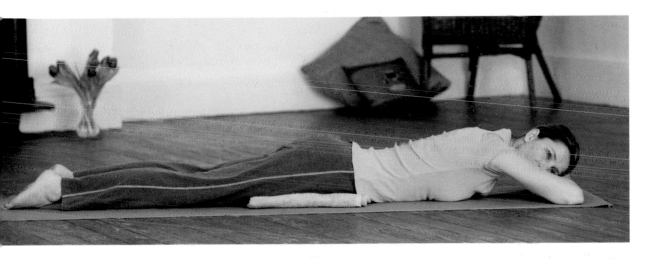

⊛ How to do it

1. Lie on your abdomen, with a flat cushion or folded towel under your hips. (This discourages accentuation of the spinal arch at the small of the back and so prevents back strain.) Keep your legs straight and comfortably separated.

2. Turn your head to the side. Fold your arms and rest your head on them. (You may, alternatively, rest your head on a small pillow. Bend your arms and rest them near your head.)

3. Relax your jaw and breathe in and out through your nose slowly and as fully as you can without straining. As you inhale, be aware of your abdomen making contact with the surface on which you are lying. As you exhale, sense your abdomen and chest relaxing.

4. Repeat step 3 again and again in smooth succession.

5. After a minute or two spent in contemplation of this rhythmical flow of your breath, add a visual component to enhance its calming and healing effects. With each inhalation, picture an intake not only of life-enriching oxygen, but also of other nourishing substances. With each exhalation, imagine the expulsion not only of metabolic wastes, but also of noxious agents that produce pain, fatigue and suffering. Let each exhalation deepen your relaxation.

6. When you are ready to get up, ease yourself onto your hands and knees and sit on your heels. You can move easily into the Pose of a Child (page 108), or turn onto your side and get up safely (page 64).

POSE OF A CHILD (YOGAMUDRA)

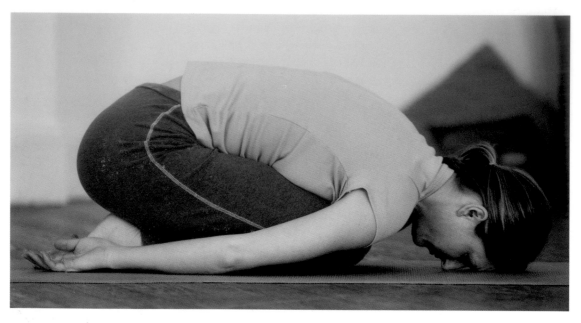

⊕ What it does

▸ Promotes all-over relaxation.

▸ While you are breathing regularly in this posture, your internal organs receive a gentle massage which enhances their circulation and also the elimination of wastes.

▸ Helps to keep the spine flexible.

▸ Eases pressure on nerves branching off the spine.

⊛ How to do it

1. Sit on your heels, as in the Firm Posture (page 20). Relax your jaw and breathe regularly.

2. Slowly bend forwards and rest your forehead on the mat, or on a pillow on the mat. You may, alternatively, turn your head to the side. Relax your arms and hands beside you, with your palms turned upwards.

3. Stay in this posture for as long as you are comfortable doing so. Breathe slowly and smoothly.

4. Slowly sit up and resume your starting position.

⊘ Note

This is an excellent counter posture to perform after backward-bending exercises such as the Bow (page 52), the Cobra (page 86) and the Camel (page 104).

▽ Variation

1. Sit on your heels but separate your knees between a bolster.

2. Bend forwards and let the bolster support your weight; wrap your arms around it.

3. Stay in this posture for as long as you are comfortable while breathing regularly.

4. Slowly sit up.

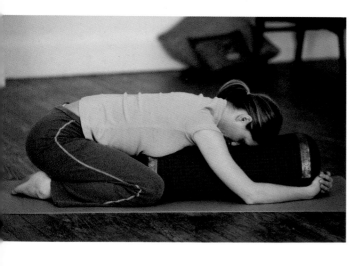

PALMING THE EYES

⊕ What it does
▸ Relaxes tired eye muscles and helps to prevent eyestrain.
▸ Reduces tension build up in face and body.
▸ Enhances concentration.

⊛ How to do it
1. Sit at a desk or table where you can rest your elbows. Vigorously rub your palms together a few times to warm them.
2. Gently place your palms, with fingers together, over closed eyes. Do not put pressure on your eyeballs. Relax your jaw and breathe regularly throughout the exercise.
3. Stay in this position for about two minutes to start with; longer if you have time and are comfortable doing so. With each exhalation, relax a little more.
4. When you are ready to end the exercise, separate your fingers to gradually re-introduce light. Open your eyes.
5. Relax your arms and hands.
6. You may blink your eyes several times to lubricate them with natural moisture.

⊘ Notes
• *Computer users are encouraged to practise Palming during short breaks from routine work to help counteract the impact of glare on the eyes.*
• *Motorists will welcome a break to rest their eyes during long road trips. Park your vehicle safely, rest your elbows on your steering wheel and practise Palming.*
• *While palming your eyes you can also practise Rhythmic Diaphragmatic Breathing (page 53), Anti-Anxiety Breath (page 60) or Pursed-Lip Breathing (page 54) for added benefits.*

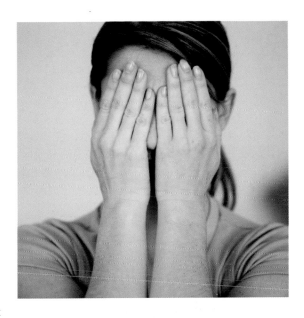

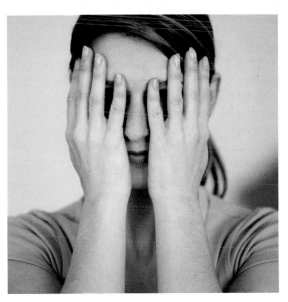

Sleep Disturbances

Sleep disturbances affect many people, and the elderly and those with psychiatric disorders, such as major depression, may be particularly prone to them.

Of these disturbances, insomnia (sleeplessness) is the most prevalent. Others include difficulty falling asleep; difficulty sleeping at night or other preferred sleep time; awakening earlier than desired; excessive daytime sleepiness; and nocturnal events such as nightmares and sleepwalking.

Numerous factors contribute to sleep disturbances. They include such factors as a change in one's sleeping environment; doing shift work; pain, anxiety or depression; various illnesses including those causing breathing problems (pages 50–51) and urinary difficulties (page 73).

The consequences of disturbed sleep include: impaired concentration, judgement and memory; likelihood of accidents; higher risk of illness; and reduced productivity. All of these impact on quality of life.

Sleep apnoea syndrome

This is characterized by a cessation of breathing during sleep, for 10 seconds or longer, occurring at least five times per hour. It may be due to an obstruction or to a central nervous system (CNS) disorder.

In obstructive sleep apnoea, movement of the diaphragm and chest muscles is apparent but not effective against a partial obstruction, as indicated by snoring. As oxygen intake decreases, the person awakens to breathe. Frequent awakenings disrupt the normal sleep cycle.

Sleep apnoea tends to be high among people in certain occupations, such as long-distance lorry (truck) drivers. The condition is worsened by obesity (page 113), which further obstructs the airways that relax and become narrow during sleep.

Sleep hygiene

The following measures may help to prevent sleep disturbances and promote refreshing slumber:

• Establishing a regular bedtime and wake-up time.

• Regular daily exercise, but avoiding vigorous exercise too close to bedtime.

• Taking measures to counteract anxiety (page 78) and to promote calm before going to sleep.

• Avoiding tobacco, alcohol and caffeinated drinks close to bedtime.

• Taking measures to avoid being overweight (page 113).

CAT STRETCH

⊕ What it does

▸ Reduces tension build up and promotes relaxation.
▸ Facilitates deep breathing and therefore enhances oxygenation of all the body's tissues.
▸ Gives a therapeutic stretch to muscles of the arms, legs and torso.
▸ Improves circulation throughout the body.
▸ Keeps the spine flexible.

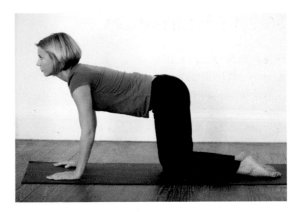

⊛ How to do it

1. Get on your hands and knees. Relax your jaw and breathe regularly.
2. On an exhalation, lower your head and tuck your hips down so that your back becomes rounded.
3. Hold the posture for a few seconds while breathing regularly.
4. Inhale and resume your starting position.
5. On a subsequent inhalation, carefully tilt your head backwards and raise and stretch out one leg.
6. Hold the posture for a few seconds while breathing regularly.
7. Resume your starting position.
8. Repeat steps 5 to 7 with the other leg.
9. On an exhalation, lower your head, bend one leg and bring the knee towards your forehead.
10. Hold the posture for a few seconds while breathing regularly.
11. Resume your starting position.
12. Repeat steps 9 to 11 with the other leg.
13. Repeat the entire sequence (steps 2 to 12) as many times as you wish in slow succession.
14. Sit on your heels and rest, or relax in the Pose of a Child (page 108).

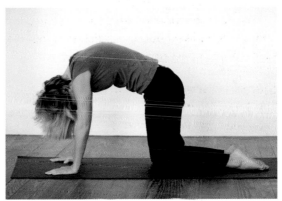

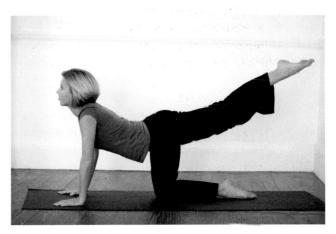

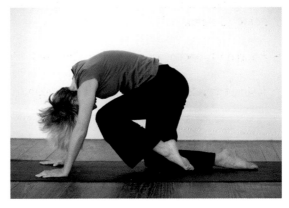

BREATH COUNTING

⊕ What it does

▸ Inspired by Zen masters, this seemingly simple breathing exercise is in fact very effective in calming the body and soothing the nerves. It diverts your attention from disturbing environmental stimuli and everyday concerns, bringing a sense of stillness that is conducive to deep relaxation.

⊛ How to do it

1. Sit tall in any comfortable position (see pages 19–21) Relax your jaw and breathe regularly. Close your eyes.
2. On an exhalation, mentally count "one".
3. Inhale.
4. On the next three exhalations, count "two", "three" and "four", in sequence.
5. Repeat steps 3 and 4 again in smooth succession. Gradually increase practice time as you become more familiar and comfortable with the technique.
6. Open your eyes and get up slowly (page 64).

Note

⊘ *You will know that your attention has strayed when you find yourself counting higher than four. Simply start again from one. Do not be discouraged if this happens often at first. Be patient and persevere.*

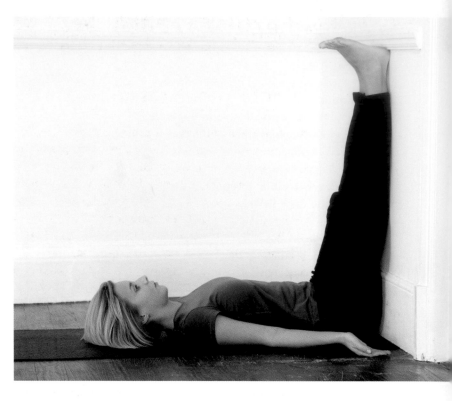

LEGS UP (VIPARITA KARANI)

⊕ What it does

▸ **Soothes the nervous system. Promotes harmony and deep relaxation of body and mind.**

⊛ How to do it

1. Bend your legs and carefully manoeuvre your body so that by raising your legs you can rest your feet, one at a time, against the wall.
2. Ease your bottom close to the wall so that your legs are straight up and form a 90-degree angle with your torso. Relax your arms a little away from your sides. Close your eyes.
3. As you inhale slowly, smoothly and as deeply as you comfortably can, imagine bringing into your system peace, refreshment and healing, or any other positive qualities you desire.
4. As you exhale slowly and as thoroughly as you can without strain, visualize banishing from your system tension, anxiety and fatigue, or any other negative qualities. Use your exhalation to let your body sink more deeply into the floor.
5. Repeat steps 4 and 5 again and again in smooth succession.
6. When you are ready to get up do so slowly and carefully: bend your legs, ease them back onto the floor and get up safely (page 64).

Caution

① *Omit this posture if you have recently formed blood clots in your veins.*

Weight problems

In an age of fizzy drinks, fast food and ready meals, packed with sugar and added fat, there are an increasing number of people with serious weight problems. If you weigh 10 to 20 percent more than the weight considered normal for your height, build, sex and age, you may be regarded as overweight.

If you are more than 20 percent above your "desirable" weight according to the above criteria, you are officially considered to be obese.

Obese people have an increased risk of developing heart disease, high blood pressure (page 61), breathing disorders (page 50), diabetes, gallbladder disease and sleep apnoea (page 110). When obesity is associated with a high-fat diet, the risk of breast, colon and prostate cancer increases.

In order to shed unwanted weight and keep it off, the experts suggest that you should strive to become healthy, rather than just thin. To achieve this, there is perhaps no better long-term measure than a combination of eating nutritiously and exercising regularly.

The benefits of regular exercise include: burning excess calories by speeding up metabolism, building muscle (people with more muscle burn more calories), boosting self-esteem and relieving stress.

In addition to the above benefits, exercise reduces the risk of certain diseases developing and it can also help alleviate depression and mood swings.

CHAIR TWIST (BHARADVAJASANA)

⊕ **What it does**

▸ Permits torsion (twisting) of the spine on both sides, giving a therapeutic massage to nerves branching off the spinal column.
▸ Keeps the spine flexible.
▸ Tones the lower back muscles.
▸ Tones transverse and oblique abdominal muscles.
▸ Enhances circulation in the kidney area, at the small of the back.
▸ Revitalizes the adrenal glands, situated atop the kidneys. (Almost all body systems are influenced by adrenal gland hormones.)
▸ Aids digestion and combats constipation.

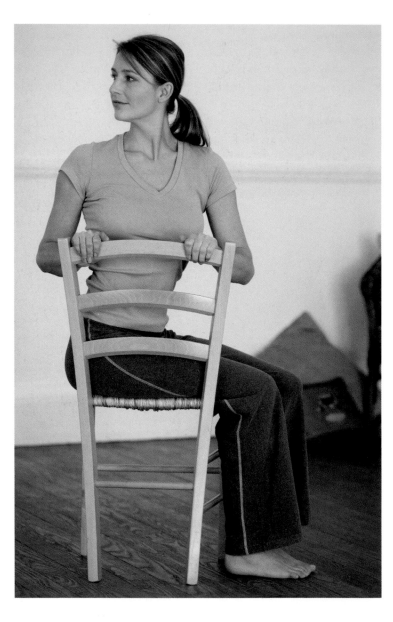

⊛ **How to do it**

1. Sit sideways on a straight-backed chair with no arms, with the back of the chair on your right. Rest your feet, comfortably separated, flat on the floor. Check that you are sitting tall. Relax your jaw and breathe regularly.
2. On an exhalation, slowly twist your upper body to the right, keeping your lower body as still as you can. Hold on to the chair back with both hands. Look towards your right shoulder.
3. Hold the posture for as long as you can with absolute comfort while breathing regularly.
4. Inhale and slowly untwist to resume your starting position. Relax your arms and hands.
5. Change your position so that you are now sitting with the back of the chair on your left.
6. Exhale and twist your upper torso to the left. Hold on to the chair back with both hands. Look towards your left shoulder.
7. Hold the posture for as long as you can with absolute comfort while breathing regularly.
8. Inhale and slowly untwist. Relax your arms and hands.

MOUNTAIN POSTURE (PARVATASANA)

⊕ What it does

▸ Facilitates deep breathing, through which the body's cells receive oxygen.

▸ Promotes good circulation, through which tissues receive nutrients.

▸ Tones pelvic, back and abdominal muscles.

▸ Discourages fat deposits around the waist and abdomen.

▸ Improves muscular support for internal organs.

▸ Tones chest and arm muscles.

⊛ How to do it

1. Sit tall on a chair (see page 21). Relax your jaw and breathe regularly.

2. Inhale and stretch your arms overhead, keeping them close to your ears. Press your palms together if you can.

3. Hold the posture for several seconds while breathing regularly. Increase the holding time as you become more familiar with the technique.

4. Exhale and lower your arms. Rest.

⊘ Note

You may do this exercise while sitting on a mat, with your legs folded (page 19) or in the Firm Posture (page 20).

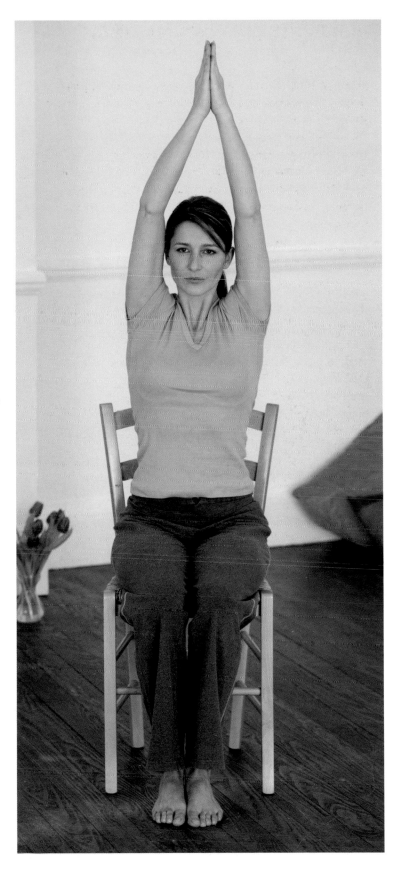

STICK POSTURE (YASTIKASANA)

⊕ What it does
▸ Gives a therapeutic stretch to the whole body.
▸ Discourages fat build up at the midriff.
▸ Facilitates deep breathing for a better oxygen intake.

⊼ How to do it
1. Stand tall with your weight equally distributed between your feet. Relax your jaw and breathe regularly.
2. Inhale and stretch your arms overhead. Keep them close to your ears. Bring your palms together if you can.
3. Hold the stretch for as long as you comfortably can while breathing regularly.
4. Exhale and lower your arms. Rest.

⊘ Note
See page 68 for a lying version of this posture.

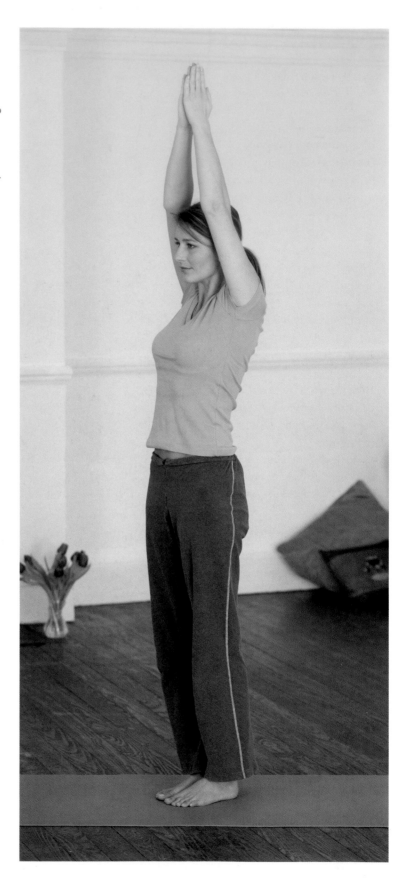

HALF MOON (ARDHA CHANDRASANA)

⊕ What it does

▸ Conditions muscles of the abdomen that are often underexercised.
▸ Tones back muscles.
▸ Keeps the spine flexible.
▸ Discourages fat build up at the midriff.
▸ Facilitates deep breathing.
▸ Keeps the shoulder joints moving freely and prevents stiffness.
▸ Tones arm muscles.

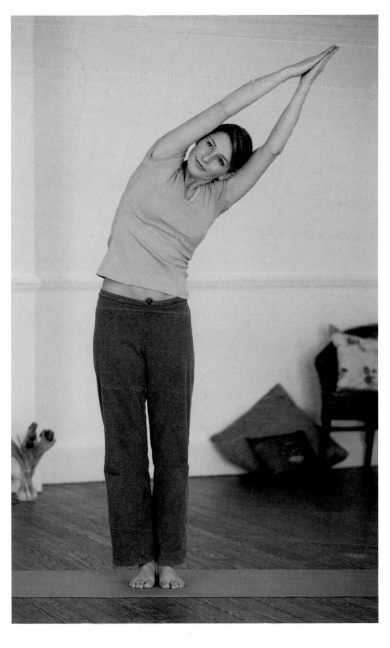

⊛ How to do it

1. Stand tall with your feet close together. Relax your arms at your sides. Relax your jaw and breathe regularly.
2. Inhale and bring your arms straight overhead. Keep them close to your ears. Bring the palms together if you can.
3. On an exhalation, slowly and smoothly bend your upper body to one side, as far as you comfortably can.
4. Hold this sideways stretch for a few seconds but keep breathing regularly.
5. Inhale and resume your starting position. Relax your arms. Rest briefly.
6. Repeat the exercise on the other side (steps 2 to 5).

ALTERNATE NOSTRIL BREATHING (NADI SHODHANAM)

⊕ What it does

▸ There is, in health, a predictable alternating of breath between the right and left nostrils. For about two hours, breathing is predominantly through one nostril and then it shifts to the other. This is a natural biological rhythm.

▸ A persisting blockage of one nostril with air flow through the other for more than a few hours can be a sign of impending ill health. Such a state can be precipitated by various occurrences, including: emotional upsets, sleep disturbances, nutritional deficits and infection.

▸ By deliberately changing the flow of air from one nostril to the other in a regular fashion, Alternate Nostril Breathing helps to maintain or to restore the natural metabolic rhythm: a balance between the building up (anabolic) and breaking down (catabolic) processes that together constitute metabolism, which is the sum of all the physical and chemical changes that take place in the body.

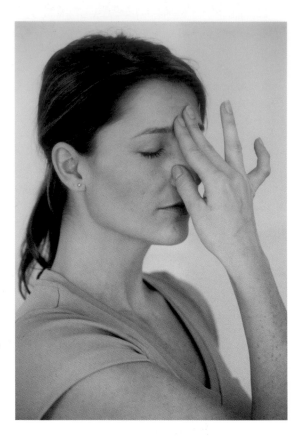

⊛ How to do it

1. Sit tall in any comfortable position. Relax your jaw and breathe regularly.
2. Rest your left hand in your lap or knee. With your right hand raised in front of you, arrange the fingers as follows: fold the two middle fingers towards the palm (or rest them lightly on the bridge of the nose once the exercise is in progress). You will use your thumb to close off the right nostril, and your ring finger (or ring and little fingers) to close off your left nostril.
3. Close your eyes. Using your thumb, close your right nostril and inhale slowly and as deeply as you can through your left nostril.
4. Close your left nostril, releasing closure of the right and exhale slowly and completely through your right nostril.
5. Inhale through your right nostril.
6. Close your right nostril and release closure of the left. Exhale. This completes one round of Alternate Nostril Breathing.

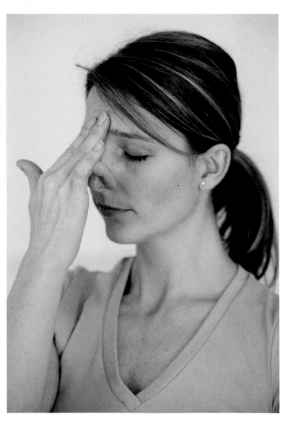

Allergies

The word "allergy" is derived from the Greek "allos" which means other and "ergon" which means work. It describes a hypersensitive reaction to a foreign substance (allergen) by the body's immune system. The reaction may be due to the release of histamine or histamine-like substances from injured cells.

Common allergens include: house dust, cigarette smoke, animal dander, pollens and insect venom.

An allergic reaction may take many forms, including rashes, nasal congestion, asthma, hay fever and ear and eye irritations.

Stresses such as inadequate diet, emotional upsets, insufficient sleep, infections and the use of certain drugs can precipitate an allergic response.

Drug allergies

Among the drugs most likely to cause allergic reactions are: sulfas, barbiturates, anticonvulsants, insulin and local anaesthetics.

Signs and symptoms of allergic reactions to drugs include: difficulty breathing, wheezing, rash, hives and generalized itching.

Food allergies

Notable among the foods that cause allergies are the proteins in cow's milk, egg whites, peanuts, wheat and soybeans. Other foods that can cause problems include beans, berries, corn and shellfish. Yellow food dye No. 5 may also produce an allergic response.

Signs and symptoms of food allergies include nausea or vomiting, abdominal pain, diarrhoea, eczema, swelling beneath the skin, hives, swelling of the lips, eyes, tongue, face or throat and nasal congestion.

HALF SHOULDERSTAND (ARDHA SARVANGASANA)

⊕ **What it does**

▸ Enhances the blood supply to nervous structures within the head.

▸ Counteracts the downward pull of gravity by relieving congestion in the body's lower structures.

▸ Tones the muscles of the neck, back and abdomen.

▸ Revitalizes the organs within the trunk and enhances the circulation and functioning of the lymphatic, nervous and endocrine systems.

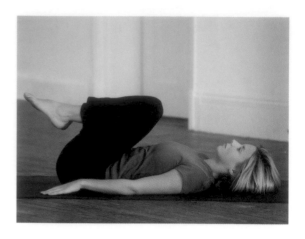

🧍 **How to do it**

1. Lie on your back with your legs stretched out in front and your arms at your sides. Relax your jaw and breathe regularly throughout the exercise.
2. Bring one bent knee then the other to your chest.
3. Straighten one leg at a time to point your feet upwards.
4. Exhale and kick backwards with both feet at once to bring your hips off the mat. Support your hips with your hands.
5. Maintain this posture for as long as you are comfortable in it, while breathing regularly.
6. To come out of the posture, rest your hands on the mat, close to your body. Keep your head pressed to the mat and very slowly lower your torso, from top to bottom, onto the mat.
7. Bend your knees, stretch out your legs one at a time and rest.

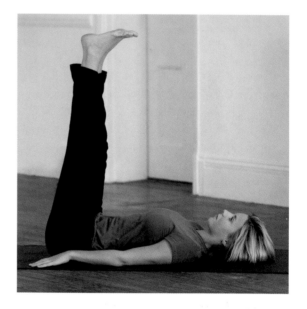

! **Caution**

Do not practise this posture during your menstrual period. Omit it from your exercise programme if you have an ear or eye disorder, high blood pressure, heart disease or other cardiovascular disorder. Check with your doctor.

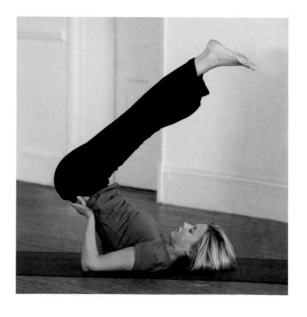

FULL SHOULDERSTAND (SARVANGASANA)

⊕ What it does

▸ The benefits derived from the Full Shoulderstand are the same as for the Half Shoulderstand. In addition, the Full Shoulderstand, through the contraction of muscles at the front of the neck, combined with gentle pressure of chin on chest, has a regulating effect on the thyroid gland. (Improved thyroid function benefits the entire human organism.)

⊛ How to do it

1. Lie on your back with your legs stretched out in front and your arms at your sides. Relax your jaw and breathe regularly.
2. Bring one bent knee then the other to your chest.
3. Straighten one leg at a time to point your feet upwards.
4. Exhale and kick backwards with both feet at once to bring your hips off the mat. Support your hips with your hands.
5. Gradually move one hand at a time towards your upper back until your body is vertical. Your chin should be in contact with your chest.
6. Hold the posture for as long as you are comfortable in it while breathing regularly.
7. To come out of the posture, tilt your legs slightly backwards. Rest your arms on the mat beside your torso. Keep your head pressed to the mat and slowly lower your body, from top to bottom, to the mat. Bend your knees, stretch out your legs one at a time and rest.

① Caution

These are the same as for the Half Shoulderstand. In addition, omit the Full Shoulderstand if you suffer from neck pain.

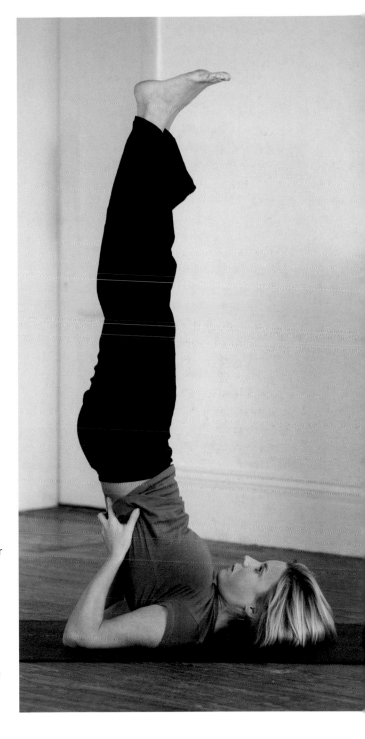

TONGUE CLEANSING

⊕ **What it does**

▸ Counteracts the effects of breathing through the mouth, which makes the oral membranes dry and vulnerable to infection.

▸ Helps to keep the breath fresh.

▸ Helps to avert a sore throat or prevent it from worsening.

⊛ **How to do it**

1. You need a metal teaspoon (or a special tongue scraper, available at stores that sell yoga supplies). A toothbrush is not recommended.

2. On an exhalation, stick out your tongue as far as you comfortably can. Use the concave side of the spoon to scrape away, from back to front, deposits accumulated on the tongue. Do so firmly but gently.

3. Inhale, pull in your tongue and close your mouth. Breathe regularly.

4. Rinse away the deposits on the spoon under cold running water.

5. Repeat steps 2 to 4 once or twice.

6. Finish by thoroughly rinsing your mouth and perhaps also brushing and flossing your teeth.

7. Clean the teaspoon with soap and water, dry it and put it away for future use.

EYE SPLASHING

⊕ **What it does**

▸ **Cleanses the eyes.**

▸ **Useful in relieving itching and other allergic eye symptoms.**

▸ **Reduces tension buildup in the eye muscles; soothes and relaxes the eyes and counteracts eyestrain.**

⊛ **How to do it**

1. Put clean, cool water in a clean basin.

2. Bend over the basin and, with clean hands, gently splash water into your open eyes a few times.

3. Gently pat your closed eyes with a clean, soft towel to dry them.

4. Rest for a minute or two with your eyes closed. Relax your jaw and breathe regularly.

NASAL WASH (NETI)

⊕ **What it does**

▸ Keeps the nasal passages clear and soothes their mucous lining.

▸ Increases the tolerance of the nasal mucous membrane to irritants.

▸ Promotes physiological harmony by enabling you to breathe freely through the nostrils.

⊛ **How to do it**

1. Dissolve one-quarter of a teaspoon of salt in a cup of warm water (the approximate concentration of sodium in blood and tissue fluids).

2. Pour a little of the solution into a clean cupped hand. Close one nostril with a thumb or finger and very carefully inhale some of it into the open nostril.

3. Briskly, but not forcefully, breathe out to expel the fluid into a wash-basin or other receptacle.

4. Repeat the procedure with the same nostril once or twice.

5. Repeat the procedure two or three times with the other nostril. Breathe normally and rest.

⊘ **Note**

Special neti pots are available in stores that sell yoga supplies.

FISH POSTURE (MATSYASANA)

⊕ What it does

▸ Expands the chest to facilitate deep breathing for better oxygen delivery to all tissues.

▸ Enhances the functioning of internal organs by stretching and toning torso muscles, and also through a gentle internal massage.

▸ Stimulates the thymus gland and so contributes to the competence of the immune system.

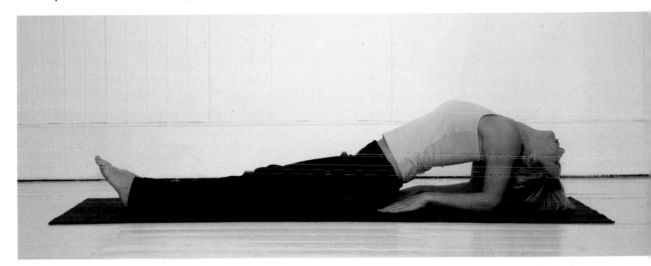

⊛ How to do it

1. Lie on your back with your legs stretched out in front and your arms at your sides. Relax your jaw and breathe regularly.
2. Bend your arms and press on your elbows to help you to raise your chest and arch your back.
3. Very carefully stretch your neck and ease your head towards your shoulders. Gently rest the top of your head on the mat. (Take most of the weight on your bottom and elbows; not on your head.)
4. Hold this posture for a few seconds to start with; longer as you become more comfortable with it. Breathe slowly, smoothly and as deeply as you can without straining
5. Very carefully ease yourself out of the posture to resume your starting position. Rest.

⊘ Note

The Knee Hug (page 39) is a good posture to do following the Fish.

⊙ Cautions

• *Omit this posture during the first three days of menstruation.*
• *Omit it if you have neck pain or suffer from a balance disorder such as vertigo or dizziness.*
• *If you have a thyroid gland problem, first check with your doctor if you plan to include this posture in your exercise programme.*

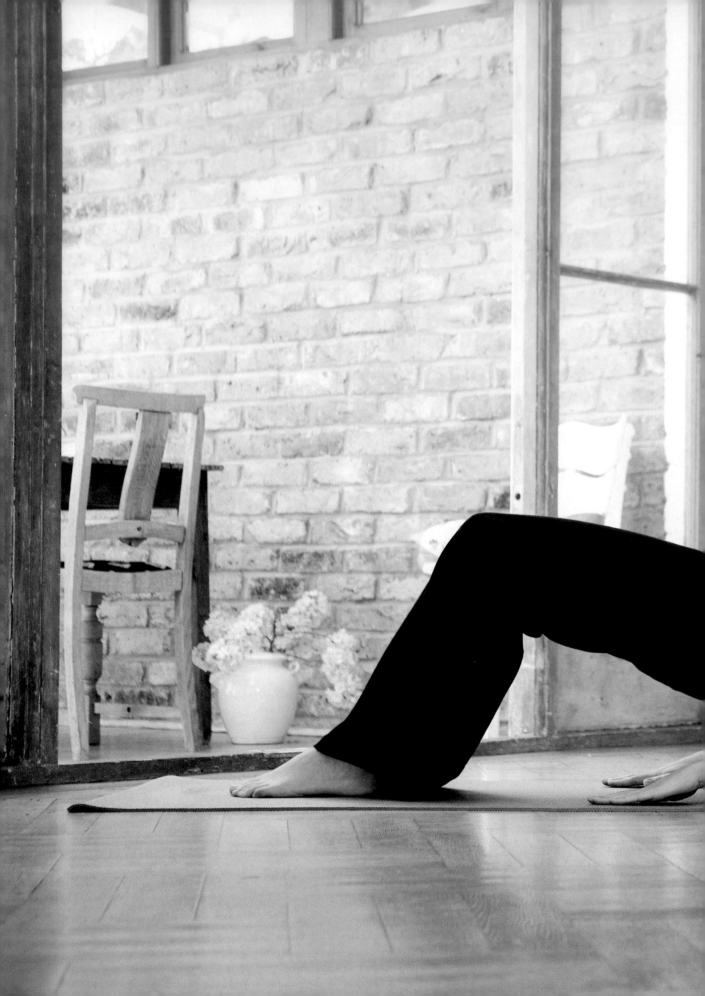

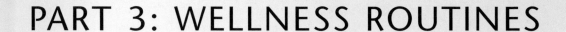

PART 3: WELLNESS ROUTINES

Wellness may be regarded as a state that reflects an individual's integrated efforts to function optimally. Health, according to the World Health Organization, is a "state of complete physical, mental and social wellbeing and not merely the absence of disease or infirmity." This state of equilibrium is not static, however, and it is normal for it to be disturbed when conditions change.

The tendency among health-care professionals has been to focus on disease rather than wellness, probably because their training emphasized the treatment of disease rather than the prevention of illness.

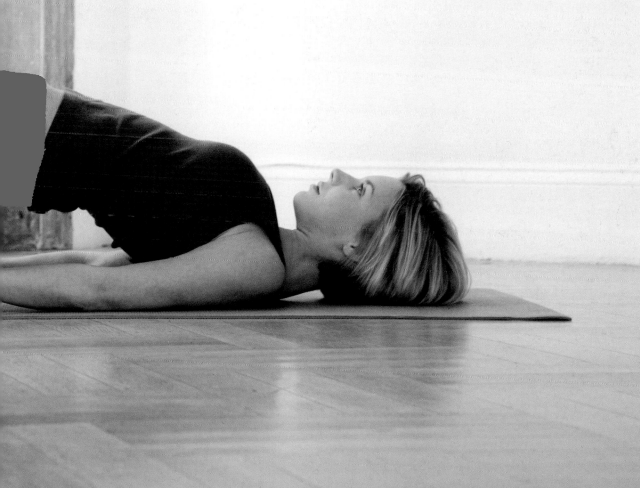

The yoga approach

Yoga takes a different approach. It encourages and supports the attaining and maintaining of wellness, in which body, mind and spirit work together in harmony. Its goal is essentially that of prevention: stopping the development and progression of disease by boosting the performance of the body's healing system. It does this by providing the "tools" and teaching the skills for developing and practising healthy lifestyle behaviours, so as to strengthen body and mind and enhance immunity to disease. Prevention is always better than cure.

Although some illnesses will occur despite our best efforts to prevent them, others are far from inevitable. Osteoporosis (page 40), for example, can largely be prevented through early attention to a balanced diet and regular exercise. Repetitive Strain Injury (page 46) can also be averted in many cases by practising good posture and body mechanics and taking periodic breaks for doing stress-relieving exercises. And in those conditions that threaten free movement, as in some forms of arthritis (page 30), good nutrition and regular exercise can do a great deal to delay or even avert impaired mobility.

Wellness requires attention and effort. It is a result of maintaining a healthy lifestyle such as good diet, exercise and implementing stress-reduction strategies. It also entails being mindful of the spiritual, or non-physical, component of the whole person, which meditative practices help to nurture.

Yoga routines

The routines that follow will help you in your endeavours to maximize your potential to function at your personal best. They are holistic in orientation, allowing you an opportunity to attend not only to the physical body (through the asanas, or postures), but also to the non-physical components of your healing system (through pranayama, or breathing exercises, and by means of imagery and other forms of meditation).

The programmes offered are designed to make the transition from one exercise to the next as logical and easy as possible. Do, however, feel completely free to modify the order in which they are given to suit your own special needs and preferences.

The routines have also been created so as to provide stretching and strengthening for the body's major muscle groups with economy of movement to prevent fatigue, to keep joints moving freely, to enhance your ability to concentrate and to facilitate efficient breathing.

Before starting to put any of the routines into practice, you may find it useful to review Part 2, particularly the Precautions (pages 16–17).

20-MINUTE WORKOUT FOR MEN AND WOMEN

If you are reasonably fit and have no disability, you will find this routine quite manageable. Do it at least every other day, to help you to build upon and maintain your current level of fitness.

This routine is also suitable for weekend practice, when you may have a little more time than during the week. The number of repetitions suggested may be modified to suit your particular needs.

START WITH:

1. Dynamic Cleansing Breath 10 to 30 times | *page 87*

WARM UPS:

1. Infinity Neck Stretches 3 to 5 times in each direction | *page 23*
2. Shoulder Circles 5 to 8 times in each direction | *page 23*
3. Ankle Circles 5 to 8 times in each direction, with each foot | *page 24*
4. Butterfly 10 to 20 times | *page 25*
5. Lying Pelvic Twist 5 to 8 times in each direction | *page 26*
6. Rocking Horse 5 to 10 times | *page 27*

MAIN EXERCISES:

1. Curl Up | *page 37*
2. Diagonal Curl Up | *page 37*
3. Spinal Twist | *page 96*
4. Sideways (Lateral) Stretch, sitting | *page 55*
5. Bridge | *page 38*
6. Knee Hug | *page 39*
7. Half Shoulderstand and/or Full Shoulderstand | *page 83, 84*
8. Plough | *page 85*
9. Fish | *page 57*
10. Cobra | *page 86*
11. Half Locust and/or Full Locust | *page 70, 71*
12. Bow | *page 52*
13. Pose of a Child | *page 108*
14. Tree | *page 42*

COOL DOWN AND RECOVERY:

1. Pose of Tranquillity for at least 5 minutes | *page 62–63*

ALTERNATIVE 20-MINUTE WORKOUT FOR MEN AND WOMEN

You may alternate the previous 20-minute workout with this one, to bring challenge and variety to your practice.

START WITH:

1. A minute or two of Rhythmic Diaphragmatic Breathing, sitting or lying down | *page 53*

WARM UPS:

1. Infinity Neck Stretches 3 to 5 times in each direction | *page 23*
2. Shoulder Circles 5 to 8 times in each direction | *page 23*
3. Ankle Circles 5 to 8 times in each direction, with each foot | *page 24*
4. Butterfly 10 to 20 times | *page 25*
5. Lying Pelvic Twist 5 to 8 times in each direction | *page 26*
6. Rocking Horse 5 to 10 times | *page 27*

MAIN EXERCISES:

1. Sun Salutation Series 2 to 6 sets | *page 89–91*
2. Half Moon | *page 117*
3. Eagle | *page 35*
4. Spinal Twist | *page 96*

COOL DOWN AND RECOVERY:

1. Pose of Tranquillity for at least 5 minutes | *page 62–63*

10-MINUTE WORKOUT FOR MEN AND WOMEN

When you are pressed for time, this routine, though shorter than the previous two, will give you enough of a workout to help you to maintain your health status. Try to do it at least every other day. Modify the number of repetitions suggested to suit your particular needs and circumstances.

WARM UPS:

1. Infinity Neck Stretches 3 to 5 times in each direction | *page 23*
2. Shoulder Circles 5 to 8 times in each direction | *page 23*
3. Ankle Circles 5 to 8 times in each direction, with each foot | *page 24*
4. Butterfly 8 to 12 times | *page 25*
5. Lying Pelvic Twist 5 to 8 times in each direction | *page 26*
6. Rocking Horse 5 to 8 times | *page 27*

MAIN EXERCISES:

1. Curl Up | *page 37*
2. Diagonal Curl Up | *page 37*
3. Sideways (Lateral) Stretch, sitting | *page 55*
4. Spinal Twist | *page 96*
5. Bridge | *page 38*
6. Half Locust | *page 70*
7. Pose of a Child | *page 108*
8. Angle Balance | *page 69*

COOL DOWN AND RECOVERY:

1. Legs Up, combined with imagery, for the time remaining | *page 79*

ALTERNATIVE 10-MINUTE WORKOUT FOR MEN AND WOMEN

You may alternate the previous 10-Minute Workout with this one, to bring challenge and variety to your practice.

WARM UPS:

In a standing position:
1. Infinity Neck Stretches 3 to 5 times in each direction | *page 23*
2. Shoulder Circles 5 to 8 times in each direction | *page 23*
3. Figure-Eight Wrist Rotation 5 to 8 times in each direction, with each hand | *page 24*
4. Sun Salutation Series (2 sets) | *page 89–91*

MAIN EXERCISES:

1. Stick Posture, Standing | *page 116*
2. Half Moon | *page 117*
3. Cow Head Posture, Standing | *page 34*
4. Tree | *page 42*
5. Eagle | *page 35*
6. Squatting Posture | *page 45*

COOL DOWN AND RECOVERY:

1. Pose of a Child, combined with Rhythmic Diaphragmatic Breathing, for the remaining time | *108, 53*

5-MINUTE WORKOUT FOR MEN AND WOMEN

For the busier-than-average person, who is nevertheless aware of the importance of staying fit, this 5-minute routine, along with other exercises integrated into your daily schedule, will bring cumulative benefits. The ideal is to do it every day, but failing this, try to do it every other day. Modify the number of repetitions suggested to suit your own needs and preferences.

WARM UPS:

1. Infinity Neck Stretches 3 to 5 times in each direction | *page 23*
2. Shoulder Circles 5 to 8 times in each direction | *page 23*
3. Ankle Circles 5 to 8 times in each direction, with each foot | *page 24*
4. Butterfly 5 to 10 times | *page 25*

MAIN EXERCISES:

1. Curl Up | *page 37*
2. Diagonal Curl Up | *page 37*
3. Spinal Twist | *page 96*
4. Half Locust | *page 70*
5. Pose of a Child | *page 108*
6. Stick Posture, standing | *page 116*
7. Half Moon | *page 117*

COOL DOWN AND RECOVERY:

1. Crocodile, combined with Rhythmic Diaphragmatic Breathing, for the remaining time | *page 107, 53*

ALTERNATIVE 5-MINUTE WORKOUT
FOR MEN AND WOMEN

You may alternate the previous 5-Minute Workout with this one, to bring challenge and variety to your practice.

WARM UPS:

Sitting in the Firm Posture | *page 20*
2.   Infinity Neck Stretches 3 to 5 times in each direction | *page 23*
3.   Shoulder Circles 5 to 8 times in each direction | *page 23*
4.   Figure-Eight Wrist Rotation 5 to 8 times in each direction, with each wrist | *page 24*

MAIN EXERCISES:

1.   Spinal Twist, in Firm Posture | *page 97*
2.   Sideways Stretch, in Firm Posture | *page 55*
3.   Dog Stretch | *page 58*
4.   Pelvic Stretch or Camel | *page 95, 104*

COOL DOWN AND RECOVERY:

1.   Pose of a Child, combined with Rhythmic Diaphragmatic Breathing, for the remaining time | *page 108, 53*

ESPECIALLY FOR SENIORS
(APPROXIMATELY 15 MINUTES)

This gentle routine will appeal to women and men of advancing age. It will help to ward off joint stiffness, prevent muscles from wasting and keep the circulation from becoming sluggish. Rather than feeling exhausted at the end of the session, you will feel energized.

Do the exercises every day if you can. Otherwise, try to do them every other day. Start with the smaller number of suggested repetitions and work towards the larger with each subsequent exercise session.

START WITH:

1. Sit tall on an upright chair with no armrests, that allows you to rest your feet flat on the floor. Rest your hands on your thighs or in your lap. Unclench your teeth to relax your jaw and breathe in and out of your nose slowly, smoothly and deeply as you can without straining. Spend a minute or two doing this quiet, rhythmical breathing | *page 21*

WARM UPS:

1. Infinity Neck Stretches 3 to 5 times in each direction | *page 23*
2. Shoulder Circles 3 to 5 times in each direction | *page 23*
3. Ankle Circles 3 to 5 times in each direction, with each foot | *page 24*
4. Figure-Eight Wrist Rotation 3 to 5 times in each direction, with each wrist | *page 24*

MAIN EXERCISES:

1. Mountain Posture, sitting on a chair | *page 115*
2. Chair Twist | *page 114*
3. Stick Posture, standing | *page 116*
4. Half Moon | *page 117*
5. Chest Expander | *page 59*

COOL DOWN AND RECOVERY:

1. Pose of Tranquillity in any comfortable position, with pillows placed where necessary for support and comfort. Spend at least five minutes relaxing | *page 62–63*

ANTENATAL ROUTINE (APPROXIMATELY 15 MINUTES)

Before attempting to do this routine, please check with your attending physician, obstetrician, midwife or physiotherapist. Please also review the precautions for pregnant women on page 17.

Start with the smaller number of suggested repetitions and gradually progress to the higher number. Be sensitive to your body's signals and modify these numbers to suit your own special needs.

WARM UPS:

1. Infinity Neck Stretches 3 to 5 times in each direction | *page 23*
2. Shoulder Circles 5 to 8 times in each direction | *page 23*
3. Ankle Circles 5 to 8 times in each direction, with each foot | *page 24*

MAIN EXERCISES:

Hold each posture for 3 to 5 seconds to start with, and gradually increase the holding time in subsequent exercise sessions, or make adjustments as dictated by your current condition.

1. Curl Up | *page 37*
2. Diagonal Curl Up | *page 37*
3. Pelvic Tilt, lying | *page 101*
4. Bridge | *page 38*
5. Knee Hug | *page 39*
6. Half Moon | *page 117*
7. Stick Posture, standing | *page 116*
8. Squatting Posture | *page 45*
9. Pelvic Floor Exercise combined with Rhythmic Diaphragmatic Breathing | *page 77, 53*

COOL DOWN AND RECOVERY:

1. Pose of Tranquillity in any comfortable position, for the remaining time | *page 62–63*

POSTNATAL ROUTINE (APPROXIMATELY 15 MINUTES)

Before attempting to do this routine, please check with your doctor, physiotherapist or other qualified care-giver.

Start with the smaller number of suggested repetitions and progress to the higher one as your strength and energy increase. Modify the number of repetitions as necessary. Be attentive and responsive to your body's cues.

WARM UPS:

1. Infinity Neck Stretches 3 to 5 times in each direction | *page 23*
2. Shoulder Circles 5 to 8 times in each direction | *page 23*
3. Ankle Circles 5 to 8 times in each direction, with each foot | *page 24*
4. Butterfly 8 to 12 times | *page 25*
5. Lying Pelvic Twist 4 to 6 times in each direction | *page 26*

MAIN EXERCISES:

1. Curl Up (raise only your head, at first) | *page 37*
2. Diagonal Curl Up (optional until you feel stronger) | *page 37*
3. Spinal Twist (any version) | *page 96*
4. Pelvic Tilt, lying supine or on all fours | *page 101, 103*
5. Bridge | *page 38*
6. Knee Hug | *page 39*
7. Stick Posture, lying | *page 68*
8. Half Moon | *page 117*
9. Squatting Posture | *page 45*
10. Dog Stretch | *page 58*
11. Pelvic Floor Exercise combined with Rhythmic Diaphragmatic Breathing | *page 77, 53*

COOL DOWN AND RECOVERY:

1. Crocodile (insert a flat pillow, cushion or folded towel under your hips) combined with Rhythmic Diaphragmatic Breathing and imagery | *page 107, 53*

GLOSSARY

Adrenal glands ~ Two endocrine glands located above the kidneys.

Airways ~ Natural passageways for air to and from the lungs.

Allergen ~ Any substance that produces an allergic reaction.

Anaemia ~ Deficiency in quality or quantity of red blood cells.

Anaesthetic ~ A drug causing insensitivity to touch or pain.

Analgesic ~ A remedy that relieves pain.

Antacid ~ A substance that neutralizes acid.

Antenatal ~ Occurring before birth.

Anticonvulsant ~ Agent that prevents or relieves convulsions (seizures).

Asana ~ Yoga physical exercise. A posture comfortably held.

Atrophy ~ Wasting of any part of the body.

Autonomic Nervous System (ANS) ~ The part of the nervous system that is concerned with the control of involuntary body functions. It is divided into the sympathetic and parasympathetic systems.

Body mechanics ~ The way in which you use your body and its various parts during daily activities.

Bolster ~ A firmly packed cushion, usually cylindrical in shape. Used as a support in some yoga postures.

Cardiovascular ~ Pertains to the heart and blood vessels.

Central Nervous System (CNS) ~ One of two main divisions of the nervous system, consisting of the brain and spinal cord.

Cervical ~ Pertaining to the region of the neck.

Chronic ~ Of long duration.

Coccyx ~ Terminal bone of the spinal column.

Colon ~ The large intestine, from the caecum to the rectum.

Cortisol ~ A steroid hormone. Generally described as a stress hormone.

Diaphragm ~ The dome-shaped muscular partition separating the ribcage from the abdomen. See also Pelvic diaphragm.

Diaphragmatic ~ Pertaining to the diaphragm.

Digestive tract ~ Tube from mouth to anus. It is part of the digestive system which includes the stomach and intestines.

Disc ~ See Intervertebral disc.

Diuretic ~ An agent that increases the flow of urine.

Dyspnoea ~ A distressful sensation of uncomfortable breathing that may be caused by certain heart conditions, strenuous exercise or anxiety, for example.

Endocrine gland ~ A gland whose secretion (hormone) flows directly into the bloodstream and powerfully affects various tissues.

Endorphins ~ Chemical substances produced in the brain, which have pain-relieving properties.

Extension ~ Movement that brings a limb into or towards a straight condition. Opposite of flexion.

Flexion ~ Bending a joint or limb upon itself. Opposite of extension.

Gastrointestinal tract ~ See Digestive tract.

Hamstrings ~ Three muscles on the back of the thigh. They flex the leg and adduct (bring towards the midline) and extend the thigh.

Histamine ~ A chemical substance produced when tissues are injured.

Hives ~ Itchy skin eruption. Also known as urticaria.

Hormone ~ A chemical substance that is generated in one organ and carried by the blood to another, in which it excites activity.

Hyperventilation ~ Overbreathing, as occurs in forced respiration and increased respiration.

Immune system ~ The body's natural defences against disease.

Intervertebral disc ~ Broad, flattened disc of fibrocartilage between the bodies of vertebrae.

Ligament ~ Band of fibrous tissue connecting bones that form a joint.

Lumbar ~ Refers to the loins, or part of the back between the chest and the pelvis.

Lymph ~ The fluid from blood which has passed through capillary walls to supply nutrients to tissue cells.

Lymphatic system ~ A system of vessels and glands involved in transporting lymph from the tissues to the bloodstream.

Metabolic ~ Refers to metabolism.

Metabolism ~ The sum of all physical and chemical changes that take place within an organism.

Mucous membrane ~ Membrane lining passages and cavities communicating with the air (such as the mouth and nose).

Mucus ~ Sticky fluid secreted by mucous membrane.

Musculoskeletal ~ Pertaining to the muscles and the skeleton, or the body's bony framework.

Oestrogen ~ An endocrine secretion that stimulates the female generative organs to reproductive function.

Oral ~ Pertaining to the mouth.

Oxygenation ~ Process of combining or treating with oxygen.

Parasympathetic Nervous System ~ Part of the autonomic nervous system. Its responses enhance "rest-and-digest" activities and support body functions that conserve and restore energy.

Pelvic diaphragm ~ Sling-like muscular support for the pelvic organs. Located between the legs and extends from the coccyx to the pubic bone. Also known as the pelvic floor.

Pelvic floor ~ See Pelvic diaphragm.

Physiologic ~ Refers to physiology.

Physiology ~ Study of the processes and function of the human body.

Post-natal ~ Occurring after birth.

Pranayama ~ Yoga breathing exercises. Exercises in controlled breathing.

Prone ~ Lying with the face downwards. Opposite of supine.

Psychoneuroimmunology ~ Scientific field that explores the relationship between psychological states and the immune system. The field is based on the mind–body connection and extends to the cellular level.

Quadriceps ~ A large muscle on the front of the thigh. It extends (straightens) the knee.

Respiration ~ Breathing. Inspiration and expiration.

Respiratory ~ Pertaining to respiration.

Sacral ~ Pertaining to the sacrum.

Sacroiliac joints ~ The joints formed by the hip bones and the sacrum.

Sacrum ~ A triangular bone located at the back of the pelvis. It is made up of five fused vertebrae.

Skeletal ~ Pertaining to the body's bony framework.

Sphincter ~ Circular muscle that closes a natural body opening, such as the anus.

Stressor ~ Anything that causes stress.

Supine ~ Lying on the back, with the face upwards. Opposite of prone.

Suture ~ A stitch or series of stitches used to close a wound.

Sympathetic Nervous System ~ Division of the nervous system. When activated, it produces "fight or flight" responses, including an increase in pulse and breathing rate.

Syndrome ~ A group of symptoms typical of a particular disease.

Synovial ~ Pertains to the lubricating fluid of joints.

Systemic ~ Pertaining to a whole system or collection of systems.

Tendon ~ Band of fibrous tissue forming the end of a muscle, and attaching it to a bone.

Thoracic ~ Pertaining to the chest.

Thymus ~ An endocrine gland composed of lymphoid tissue, located in the chest above the heart. It is part of the immune system.

Thyroid gland ~ A two-lobed endocrine gland situated in front of the windpipe.

Vascular ~ Pertaining to or composed of blood vessels.

Vertebra (plural, vertebrae). Any one of the 33 bones forming the spine (vertebral column).

Viscera ~ Internal organs enclosed within a cavity, especially the abdominal organs.

BIBLIOGRAPHY

American Psychiatric Association. *Diagnostic And Statistical Manual of Mental Disorders* (4th ed.). Washington, DC: American Psychiatric Association, 1994.

Anderson, Kenneth N., Anderson, Lois E., and Glanze, Walter D. (Eds.). *Mosby's Medical, Nursing, & Allied Health Dictionary* (5th ed.). St. Louis: Mosby, 1998.

Black, Joyce M., Ph.D, RN, CPSN, CCCN, CWCN, Hawks, Jane Hokanson, DNSc, MSN, RN, C, and Keene, Annabelle M., MSN, RN, C. *Medical-Surgical Nursing. Clinical Management for Positive Outcomes* (6th ed.). Philadelphia: W.B. Saunders, 2001.

Brena, Steven F., M.D. *Yoga & Medicine*. Baltimore: Penguin Books, 1972.

Carrico, Mara, and the editors of *Yoga Journal*. *Yoga Basics*. New York: Henry Holt, 1997.

Chopra, Deepak, M.D. *Quantum Healing*. New York: Bantam Books, 1989.

Doctor, Ronald M., Ph.D., and Kahn, Ada P., Ph.D. *The Encyclopedia of Phobias, Fears, and Anxieties* (2nd ed.). New York: Facts on File, 2000.

Hagen, Philip T., M.D. (Editor-in-Chief). *Mayo Clinic Guide to Self-Care*. Rochester, Minnesota: Mayo Clinic, 1999.

Hodgson, Stephen, M.D. (Editor in Chief). *Mayo Clinic on Osteoporosis*. Rochester, Minnesota: Mayo Clinic, 2003.

Hunder, Gene G., M.D. (Editor-in-Chief). *Mayo Clinic on Arthritis*. Rochester, Minnesota: Mayo Clinic, 1999.

Kendall-Reed, Penny, ND, and Reed, Stephen, MD, FRCSC. *Healing Arthritis*. Markham, Canada: Quarry Press, 2002.

King, John, M.D. (Editor in Chief). *Mayo Clinic on Digestive Health* (2nd ed.). Rochester, Minnesota: Mayo Clinic, 2004.

Krucoff, Carol, and Krucoff, Mitchell, M.D. *Healing Moves*. New York: Harmony Books, 2000.

Kuvalayananda, Swami, and Vinekar, Dr S.L. *Yogic Therapy*. New Delhi: Central Health Education Bureau, Ministry of Health, 1971.

McGilvery, Carole, Reed, Jim, Mehta, Mira, and Mehta, Silva. *The Encyclopedia of Aromatherapy, Massage and Yoga*. Enderby, England: Acropolis Books, 1994.

Noble, Elizabeth, R.P.T. *Essential Exercises for the Childbearing Year*. Boston: Houghton Mifflin, 1976.

Pascarelli, Emil, M.D., and Quilter, Deborah. *Repetitive Strain Injury. A Computer User's Guide*. New York: John Wiley & Sons, 1994.

Purna, Dr Svami. *Balanced Yoga*. Shaftesbury, Dorset: Element Books, 1992.

Quilter, Deborah. *The Repetitive Strain Injury Recovery Book*. New York: Walker and Company, 1998.

Rama, Swami, Ballentine, Rudolph, M.D., and Hymes, Alan, M.D. *Science of Breath*. Honesdale, Pennsylvania: The Himalayan International Institute of Yoga Science and Philosophy, 1979.

Shivapremananda, Swami. *Yoga for Stress Relief*. London: Gaia Books, 1997.

Siegel, Irwin M., M.D. *All about Bone: An Owner's Manual*. New York: Demos Medical Publishing, 1998.

Sparrowe, Linda, with Walden, Patricia. *The Woman's Book of Yoga & Health*. Boston & London: Shambhala, 2002.

Stuart, Gail W., PhD, RN, CS, FAAN, and Laraia, Michele T., PhD, RN, CS. *Stuart & Sundeen's Principles and Practice of Psychiatric Nursing* (6th ed.). St. Louis: Mosby, 1998.

Sutcliffe, Dr Jenny, MCSP. *Reader's Digest Body Maintenance Manual*. London: The Reader's Digest Association, 1999.

Thomas, Clayton L., M.D., M.P.H. (Ed.). *Taber's Cyclopedic Medical Dictionary* (15th ed.). Philadelphia: F.A. Davis Company, 1985.

Tortora, Gerard J., and Grabowski, Sandra Reynolds. *Principles of Anatomy and Physiology* (9th ed.). New York: John Wiley & Sons, 2000.

Weil, Andrew, M.D. *8 Weeks to Optimum Health*. New York: Alfred A. Knopf, 1997.

——. *Spontaneous Healing*. New York: Alfred A. Knopf, 1995.

Weller, Stella. *The Better Back Book*. London: Hamlyn, 2005.

——. *A Gaia Busy Person's Guide Yoga*. London: Gaia Books, 2004.

——. *Yoga Beats Asthma*. London: Thorsons, 2003.

——. *Good Housekeeping Complete Yoga*. London: HarperCollins Illustrated, 2001

——. *The Breath Book*. London: Thorsons, 1999.

——. *Pain-Free Periods* (rev. ed.). London: Thorsons, 1993.

——. *Super Natural Immune Power*. Wellingborough, England: Thorsons, 1989.

Yogendra, Smt. Sitadevi. *Yoga Simplified for Women*. Santa Cruz, Bombay: The Yoga Institute, 1972.

INDEX

Page numbers in **bold** indicate main entries for health problems. These main entries include information on the problems and the recommended exercises to help bring relief and promote healing for them.

Page numbers in *italics* indicate main entries for exercises and postures. These main entries include the benefits of the exercises, any precautions needed, and step-by-step instructions.

To my friend Kathleen Chen with affection and appreciation

First published in Great Britain in 2007 by
Collins & Brown
151 Freston Road
London
W10 6TH

An imprint of Anova Books Company Ltd.

10 9 8 7 6 5 4 3 2 1

British Library Cataloguing-in-Publication Data:
A catalogue record for this book is available from the British Library.

ISBN 1 8434 03625

Commissioning Editor: Victoria Alers-Hankey
Editor: Jane Ellis
Designer: Abby Franklin
Design Manager: Gemma Wilson
Photographer: Guy Hearn
Senior Production Controller: Morna McPherson
Models: Jennifer Young and Sandra Jones
Yoga consultant: Pagan Mace

Reproduction by Anorax Imaging Ltd
Printed by Craftprint International Ltd, Singapore

ACKNOWLEDGEMENTS

Many thanks to everyone who has contributed to this project. I am particularly grateful to:
Polly Powell for her kind referral; Victoria Alers-Hankey for a harmonious working relationship.

Special thanks go to Walter for his invaluable assistance at every stage of the project and to David for so generously sharing his computer expertise. Thanks also to Karl for his help with research and to Lora for her sincere interest.